Acclaim for Brad King and Fat Wars!

"A fascinating book. *Fat Wars* is one of the most compelling books to date on how to develop the lean body you want. Clear, concise, and scientifically sound, *Fat Wars* is a powerful guide for the path to feeling better, stronger, and leaner for life."
> —Dr. Michael A. Schmidt, Ph.D., nutritional biochemist, clinical neuroscientist, and author of *Brain Building Nutrition*

"This practical, down-to-earth book will not only tell you how to lose fat, it will help you reshape your body and permanently improve your overall health and longevity."
> —Carolyn DeMarco, M.D., physician and author of *Take Charge of Your Body: Women's Health Advisor*

"I believe Brad King has accomplished a great task with *Fat Wars*. One that has been in great need in regard to diabetes and fat management. *Fat Wars* has qualified the main reasons behind what to do or not to do in regards to obtaining a leaner, healthier, and happier life. Once a reader comprehends the message of *Fat Wars* and implements its guidelines, a life change will occur."
> —Dr. Richard H. Cockrum, President of IMMUNO-DYNAMICS, INC.

"In *Fat Wars*, Brad King has found a way to explain the true science of weight loss in a direct, engaging, and commonsense way. It is full of no-nonsense weight-loss strategies. I hope this book becomes the bible for any individual trying to lose weight or maintain their current weight."
> —Edmund R. Burke, Ph.D., professor and Director of the Exercise Science Program at the University of Colorado

"Brad King will guide you on an exciting journey to your ideal weight through the science of hormonally related nutrition and exercise. You will learn how to manage an out-of-control appetite and to bring all of your food and mood hormones into perfect balance for a leaner, healthier, happier, and longer life."
> —Sam Graci, M.A., nutritional researcher and author of *The Food Connection*

"With obesity reaching epidemic levels in the U.S., it's time to wage war. *Fat Wars* will give you all the ammunition you need to successfully fight your own battle of the bulge."
> —Ray Sahelian, M.D., bestselling author of *The Stevia Cookbook* and *Mind Boosters*

"For all those who have battled the vicious cycle of dieting and weight gain, Brad King provides a program that will guide you to a leaner, stronger body. Unlike other fat loss books, *Fat Wars'* unique approach helps you shed extra pounds, curb your appetite, and learn new exercise methods that are fun while improving the overall health of all your body systems. *Fat Wars* is not just another diet book—it is the key to permanent, healthy weight loss."
> —Lorna Vanderhaeghe, coauthor of *The Immune System Cure: Optimize Your Immune System in 30 Days—The Natural Way!*

"This book certainly helps to reaffirm our philosophy that 'Longevity Medicine promotes dying young as old as possible.'"
> —Dr. Phillip A. White, M.D., Vice President of the Canadian Longevity and Anti-Aging Academy

"Turn-up the burn and win the war. Brad King teaches the nutritional connection to optimal health hormone balance and better metabolism."
> —Michael A. Zeligs, M.D., founder of Bio Response, Boulder, Colorado, and originator of Absorbable Diindolylmethane (*Bio-Dim)

"*Fat Wars* contains one of the great secrets to long life with abundant health. Brad King takes you by the hand and guides you through to trimmer, healthier, and happier ground. The message is simple, the outcome profound."
> —Kenneth Seaton, Ph.D., D.Sc., author of *Life, Health and Longevity* and creator of the Advanced Hygiene System

"The *Fat Wars* body transformation program combines common sense with medical and physiological science. It works!"
> —Dr. Stan Gore, M.D., LL.B.

FAT WARS
action planner

BRAD J. KING

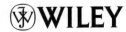

National Library of Canada Cataloguing in Publication

King, Brad J.
    Fat wars action planner / Brad J. King.

Includes bibliographical references and index.
ISBN 0-470-83250-9

    1. Weight loss. 2. Reducing diets. I. Title.

RM222.2.K563 2003   613.2'5   C2003-900098-2

Production Credits
Cover & interior text design: Interrobang Graphic Design Inc.
Printer: Tri-Graphic Printing Ltd.

Photo Credits
Cover photo: Gary Buss / Getty Images.
Author photo: Brad Stringer

Printed in Canada
10 9 8 7 6 5 4 3 2 1

CONTENTS

Preface		vii
Section I INTRODUCTION		**1**
	1. Fat Wars 101: Know Thy Enemy	11
	2. Hormones: Your Greatest Ally	17
	3. Smaller Fat People	27
	4. Waking Up Thinner	39
	5. His and Hers Designer Fat Cells	47
	6. It's All About Balance	59
	Your Body Chemistry Cheat Sheet	85
Section II FUELING YOUR BODY ON FAT WARS		**103**
Section III TRANSFORMING THROUGH BIOCIZE		**173**
	Appendix	217
	References	233
	Index	247

PREFACE

If you are reading this book right now, you're probably ready to engage in yet another battle against your wily fat cells. You may be the weary veteran of many diet and exercise plans that promised miracles and left you exhausted and disappointed—and perhaps with more body fat than you started. Or, maybe you're a burgeoning Fat Warrior: you've read and put into action the principles in my previous book, *Fat Wars: 45 Days to Transform Your Body*—and you've seen the battle against excess fat (and the health risks it poses) shift in your favour. Now, forty-five days later, you're looking for the information and guidelines you need to make those principles part of a lifelong plan. Either way, the *Fat Wars Action Planner* will arm you with the necessary weapons to finally win your personal Fat War, permanently.

When I wrote *Fat Wars*, I set out to create a guide that would help people understand how the body functions in relation to dietary intake, exercise, and the environment. I wanted to awaken readers to the fact that fat loss is a *hormonal*, *enzymatic*, and *neurochemical* process—not simply a matter of cutting calories, eating only grapefruit or only steak, and sweating it out on the treadmill. In my capacity as a nutritional researcher and fitness expert, I had received thousands of e-mails from people who had tried almost everything the diet industry had to throw at them. Some reported quick results in the form of weight loss from these programs. Others reported very limited results or none at all. But most of the people who wrote to me expressed extreme disappointment and confusion. Either they couldn't seem to lose their excess fat, or they had failed in their attempts to keep the weight off for any extended period of time. In fact, over the medium and long term, almost all of them ended up worse off than before they started.

I had dedicated years of research to exploring the reasons why almost three-quarters of our population finds it all too easy to store fat but next to impossible to lose it. I began to lecture about "Total Body Transformation" a few years ago and was taken aback by the response to these lectures. It was as if my audiences were hearing this valuable information for the very first time … and, as it turned out, they were.

I quickly learned that what people really need are easy-to-apply principles in their daily battles with the bulge. I also learned that most of the people who wrote to me or attended my lectures weren't carrying around their extra padding because of laziness or a lack of willpower. Most of them would have done just about anything to lose their excess body fat—and most of them had tried just about everything. What they lacked, however, was knowledge: an understanding of the necessary biochemical strategies that could effectively guide them through the many diet land mines they had stepped on time and again. Sadly, the vast majority of my audiences had all but given up in their attempts not only to look good again, but to improve their health and feel and perform better than they could ever imagine.

I wrote *Fat Wars: 45 Days to Transform Your Body* in response to the disappointment and confusion that reigned when it came to safe, sane, effective fat loss, and in response to that desperate need for information. I wanted readers to understand *why* they kept failing to lose body fat. Once they understood the *why*, I reasoned, they could finally learn *how* to avoid fat-loss pitfalls and instead apply proven scientific principles that would place them on the winning side—for a change.

And it worked. After the book came out, I still received e-mails, but now the content had changed. The thousands of people who became *Fat Wars* believers transformed not only their bodies, but also their overall lives. They lost excess fat, gained muscle, and reported renewed energy, better health, and a newfound confidence and pleasure in their bodies (and often their relationships). Instead of losing the battle of the bulge, they were becoming successful Fat Warriors. They began to spread the message, and *Fat Wars* became a number-one, international bestseller. A heartfelt thank you to everyone who contributed to its phenomenal success.

Fat Wars wasn't a diet book, so I didn't include recipes and eating plans. Nor was it another get-lean-quick scheme. No one needed another one of those. Rather, I wanted readers to see that, in forty-five days, they could notice a significant change—not only in appearance, but in vitality—as their metabolisms shifted from primarily fat-storing to fat-burning mechanisms. I wanted them to see and feel enough of a change to get motivated again.

It became clear, however, that readers wanted more. After the initial forty-five-day transformation period, people longed for the next step: information on how to be successful Fat Warriors for the rest of their lives. After all, it had taken years for people to become over-fat. Maintaining the edge in the Fat Wars is likewise a lifelong process.

The *Fat Wars Action Planner* is the answer to thousands of requests that sprang from the original book. It is a guide that once again explains the key concepts behind progressive transformation from over-fat to lean, but it also supplies a practical means to implement the *Fat Wars* strategies easily and consistently as part of a life plan. The *Fat Wars Action Planner* arms you with the necessary weapons to finally win your own Fat Wars. Weapons in the form of knowledge, effective eating strategies, numerous easy-to-prepare recipes and food guidelines, as well as a new scientific approach to fat-burning exercise that incorporates the original Fat Wars philosophy of "less is more" in terms of total body transformation.

The first forty-five days got you started. *The Fat Wars Action Planner* is your official guide to making total transformation a part of your life. You are about to embark on a journey to a new you. My goal is to make that journey not only highly successful but also highly enjoyable. Thousands of *Fat Wars* followers told me what they needed after the forty-five days … *The Fat Wars Action Planner* is my response. Enjoy!

ACKNOWLEDGMENTS

I wish to thank the following people for being there for me and supporting me in one way or another during the writing of *The Fat Wars Action Planner*. Without many of these people, this book may never have become a reality.

Thank you to my late mother Elva who I know is constantly watching over me. You are my angel. To Peggy Groom, I love you like a mother and I will always cherish the relationship we share. You are my earth guide. Thanks to a true humanitarian and mentor, Sam Graci, you have inspired me to be the researcher, lecturer, and health advocate I am today. To my dear friend Dr. Michael Schmidt, its amazing how you stay so humble in the face of your brilliance.

Special thanks to Susan Goldberg, I truly appreciate your level of proficiency and talent. Thanks for helping me convey my message. To one of the greatest exercise physiologists today, Jeremy Sheppard, thanks for your expertise and dedication in helping design the Biocize programs in Section III.

To one of my greatest supporters and best friends, Fred Hagadorn, thanks for always being there and offering support when I needed it most. Thanks to Deane Parkes, a man who believed in my abilities from the beginning. I will never forget that.

Most especially I want to express my gratitude to Renee, who constantly amazes me with her unending compassion, generosity, friendship and unconditional love. Thank you for being the person you are.

Finally special thanks go out to all the Fat Wars warriors of the world who came, read, became inspired and transformed their lives for the better. It is time that you gave yourselves the credit you deserve.

In order to transform ones body, you must first learn to transform your life. But in order to transform your life, you must first and foremost alter your *self-image*. Your *self-image* is like a guidance system in your life, steering you in the direction of success or failure (depending on how you see yourself).

Hypnosis is defined as the power of belief. Many of you are actually hypnotized by a false-belief, which continues to steer you towards failure. Your *self-image* guides your habits, so if you see yourself as a fat unhealthy person, then all of your actions will follow in that path — keeping you that way. When you consciously make an effort to alter your negative habits for positive ones, your self-image will eventually accept these habits as reality. Change your *self-image* and *transform yourself* into the person you deserve to be.

Here's to way beyond 45 days, here's to the rest of your life.

Wishing You Health, Happiness, and Longevity,

Brad J. King

INTRODUCTION

No Turning Back

Imagine a world where there were special health risk taxes on candy and fast food. Where doughnut boxes and chocolate-bar wrappers were printed with graphic pictures of cholesterol-clogged arteries, insulin syringes, and malignant tumors, accompanied by stern warnings that "Eating this product may cause obesity, heart disease, diabetes, high blood pressure, cancer, sexual dysfunction, pain, and depression." Imagine a world in which governments banned the advertisement of processed, sugary, fried foods and soda pop, and restricted their sale to minors in order to protect their health. Where the consumption of French fries, cupcakes, cinnamon buns, and the like was banned in public places. Where you had to show ID to buy a bag of potato chips.

Sound familiar? It should; it's how cigarette sales and smoking are dealt with by governments concerned about the health of their citizens—and about the enormous health costs associated with smoking. I'm willing to bet that most citizens support these government initiatives. After all, everybody knows that smoking kills.

But what if I told you that being over-fat was a greater risk to life and health than smoking? Would you believe me? Probably not. But according to a study by the RAND Institute in Santa Monica, California, published in the *British Journal of Public Health* in 2001, obese adults have more chronic health problems than their smoking counterparts.

What's more, the health risks associated with obesity aren't limited to just a small group. More than half of Canadians and 60% of Americans are over-fat; around one-quarter of this group is obese. Our incidence of obesity has skyrocketed by a whopping 50% in the last decade. Since 1991, obesity rates have increased throughout Canada and in every state of the United States, in both genders and across all races, age groups, and educational levels. Fat doesn't discriminate. In America, more people are overweight or obese than, collectively, smoke, or drink heavily.

Excess body fat almost always leads to a whole host of dangerous, costly health risks, and most of us don't even know it. Perhaps worse, many of us who do know it choose to ignore the facts.

Beyond Vanity: Why Losing Fat Could Save Your Life

Obesity has reached epidemic proportions in North America and beyond. In fact, the World Health Organization has classified obesity as a worldwide epidemic. And, believe me, it's much more than a cosmetic issue. Almost 300,000 people die in North America each year from conditions that are directly attributable to excess body fat and obesity. These are mortality figures one might expect from a major war, not from an age of relative peace, plenty, and prosperity. Of those that don't end up on the coroner's table, many will experience the myriad complications associated with excess fat accumulation.

What complications, you ask? Well, more than thirty known diseases can be directly linked to excess body fat, including heart disease, diabetes, high cholesterol, high blood pressure or hypertension, stroke, infertility, and cancers (including gastrointestinal, prostate, breast, and endometrial, among others). Obesity and excess fat are associated with gallbladder disease and gallstones, and immune dysfunction. They can even contribute to reproductive and sexual dysfunction (due to decreased levels of the hormone testosterone), depression, diabetes, thyroid conditions, and cardiovascular disease.

Extra fat in the neck region can close down airways during sleep, contributing to obstructive sleep apnea and other breathing problems. Let's not forget heartburn and stomach upset: excess body fat puts pressure on the one-way valve that leads from the esophagus to the stomach, which can allow acid to flow back through to the esophagus, causing heartburn. Then there are structural problems that can occur as a result of the pressures of too much weight on the frame. Many obese individuals suffer from joint-related problems such as osteoarthritis—especially in the lower back, hip, and knee areas.

The number-one killer in North America, cardiovascular disease, comes early to the over-fat, simply because their blood vessels, or microcapillaries, wear out almost three times as quickly as they do in someone who is lean. Too much body fat (especially if the majority of that fat is located in your midsection) also greatly increases the risk of developing a common middle-age condition referred to as Syndrome X, a group of health disorders that can include but are not limited to insulin resistance (the inability to properly metabolize dietary carbohydrates and sugars), abnormal blood fats (such as elevated cholesterol and triglycerides), excess body fat or obesity, and high blood pressure and heart disease. Researchers at Stanford University School of Medicine believe that poor lifestyle choices—like stress and a lack of exercise—coupled with poor nutritional habits (including a diet high in refined carbohydrates) have led to today's epidemic of this syndrome.

Excess body fat plays a huge role in the development of Type II diabetes, the most common form of the disease, which is indicated by the body's inability to manufacture or properly use the hormone insulin. The condition sets the stage for a host of diabetes-related complications, including blindness (diabetes is the leading cause of new cases of blindness in adults), kidney failure (diabetes is the leading cause of end-stage renal disease, accounting for about 40% of new cases), heart disease (the leading cause of diabetes-related deaths), and amputations.

About eighteen million North Americans have Type II diabetes. Sixteen million are U.S. citizens, about half of them undiagnosed. Every day in the United States, 2,200 new cases of diabetes are diagnosed, for an estimated total of 798,000 new cases each year. Almost 90% of Type II diabetics are over-fat; many are obese. And we're not talking adults-only any more. It's incredible to think that, a generation ago, Type II diabetes used to be known as adult-onset diabetes, because it affected adults almost exclusively. Today, the marked increase in over-fat children is mirrored by a similar increase in childhood Type II diabetes. Our kids are becoming victims of the Fat Wars, at much too early an age.

Some of the most destructive problems associated with excess body fat are not physical but psychological. Low self-esteem, depression, and eating disorders are common side effects of carrying around excess fat. The diet industry feeds right into these disorders, as people continually struggle with their frustrations and inability to lose weight and keep it off. (Regular dieting, in fact, may well encourage weight gain, a topic I'll cover in Chapter 3, Smaller Fat People).

The fatter you allow yourself to become, the greater your chances of suffering from one or more of the nasty disorders described above. The direct cost of obesity in the U.S. and Canada has been estimated at more than $100 billion per year, which makes an over-fat society everybody's business.

The saddest part is that most over-fat and obese people are likely to die before their time. If you are one of these people, your chances of reaching the estimated life expectancy of 76.7 years is, well, rather slim. Being over-fat doesn't automatically guarantee you a one-way ticket to a short life filled with disease, but it certainly increases your risk of being one of the statistics.

Food: The Real Scoop!

The opening scenario is a crude metaphor, but it's also a wake-up call: we need to take a close look at what we eat and how it affects our health and well-being. Unfortunately, analyzing the true value of the foods we eat is often easier said than done.

While it's a sad fact that the overweight and obese are often shunned in our image-conscious society, the foods that make us over-fat are accepted parts of North American life. In fact, they're woven into our national consciousness—as Canadian as back bacon or maple syrup, American as apple pie. Criticizing the average citizen's eating habits is downright unpatriotic.

And then there's the food itself. Very few of us ever associate our myriad less-than-optimal food choices with ill health. How can anything that looks, tastes, and smells so great be *that* bad for you? Here, food processing is culpable: the manufacturers of so-called convenience and fast foods hook us by targeting our most sensitive senses—taste and smell. They use a range of sophisticated techniques to make their products as appetizing as possible. What we don't see is the mimicry: the foreign, toxic compounds we call preservatives, artificial flavor enhancers, moisturizers, coloring agents, fungus retardants, and hydrogenated fats.

I'm not talking about only the more obvious junk food like candy, chips, soda pop, or fast food, although they're certainly part of the problem. A large percentage of food we've come to think of as good for us has been refined to the point where anything of nutritional value disappears. Take something as basic as wheat. It used to offer many nutrients for optimal health. Modern processing into white flour, however, has stripped out the vitamins, minerals, hull, germ, fiber, and seed—all nutrients the body thrives on. We are left with a shadow food, whose nutrients have been replaced with a variety of chemical compounds that slowly erode our cells and contribute to ill health and obesity. Most of these processed wonders, which look so good on the shelf, end up taking much more from the body than they give!

And the news keeps getting worse. New research presented in the *Journal of Lipid Research* in 2002 indicates that unwanted weight gain (excess body fat) may also be strongly linked to hormone-disrupting contaminants. In this case, a common synthetic estrogen, called Bisphenol A or BPA, both triggers and stimulates two of the key biological mechanisms underlying obesity: first, it increases the number of fat cells (hyperplasia), and second, it enhances their fat storage abilities (fat cell hypertrophy). The scariest thing of all is that BPA is a polycarbonate plastic used as cavity-preventing coating for children's teeth, a coating in metal cans to prevent contact with food contents, as the plastic in food containers, refrigerator shelving, baby bottles, returnable containers for juice, milk, and water, microwave ovenware, and eating utensils. Microwave heating with polycarbonate plastics can also leach BPA into the food source.

If you don't think your food or container choices have any profound impact on your future, think again. As we learn more and more about the human body and its interactions with its environment, it becomes ever more apparent that your lifestyle and dietary choices are likely far more important to your health than your genetic makeup. Many scientists would agree that the choices you make every day determine up to 80% of your health status—less than 20% of our ailments are genetically ordained. In his groundbreaking book, *Genetic Nutritioneering*, Jeffrey Bland, Ph.D., explains that our genetic inheritance (or genotype) is little more than a template upon which we build our unique life experience. While our genetic codes may be fixed, their expression (or phenotype) changes constantly, adapting to diet, lifestyle, and environment. To a very large extent, it's up to you whether you choose to express your genes toward health or disease—and toward obesity or leanness.

Don't Weight for Me!

Okay, so you've accepted that excess fat and obesity are problems of epidemic proportions in our society. And you're well aware of the health risks that accompany this epidemic. But how are you supposed to gauge whether you're at risk? Here's one way *not* to judge yourself: the scale alone.

We are a society completely infatuated with weight. We watch our weight—like hawks. We gauge our success or failure on any weight-loss program by our bathroom scales. And, when the numbers become unacceptably high, we cry out, "I have to lose some weight!"

What we really should be saying is, "I have to lose some fat!"

The difference is subtle yet profound. We have been taught to lump all weight into the same category. But not all weight is created equal! The body is comprised of lean tissues (skeletal, blood, organ, muscle) and body fat. Muscle weighs up to four times more than fat does, even though it takes up less space. And as you will learn throughout the *Fat Wars Action Planner*, muscle can either make you or break you in the Fat Wars. This is because muscle dictates the rate at which you can burn calories at rest by raising your metabolism. In other words, the more muscle you maintain or grow (yes, even for you women), the more fat you can burn naturally, even while you're resting.

Body fat, on the other hand, is inert. In other words, as many of you know too well, it just sits there. Its main function is to act as a reserve tank for calories. Unfortunately, many people never learn how to successfully access these storage tanks—so their fat cells just keep getting larger. The problem is exacerbated (as you will learn) by the fact that the larger these fat cells become, the harder it is to maintain your muscle mass.

North Americans spend more than $33 billion annually on weight-loss products and services. Right now, one-third of women and one-quarter of men are either starting or finishing the latest fad diet. Too bad nobody told them that only 5% of dieters are successful at keeping the weight off after a two-year period. One plausible reason so many diets fail is that the majority of them on the market do not support lean tissue (muscle). Consequently the majority of the weight lost on them comes from this valuable source. If would-be Fat Warriors focused on *losing fat* as opposed to simply *losing weight* in the form of lean body tissues (especially muscle), there would be a lot more diet success stories out there.

Some kinds of weight are much healthier for you than others. Instead of focusing on losing weight, focus on losing body fat—not muscle. In the following pages, I'll show you how to win the Fat Wars by doing just that.

So, if the number on the scale isn't the most reliable way of assessing whether the amount of fat you're carrying puts you at risk for health problems, what is? The answer is simple: your overall body-fat percentage, or the proportion of your total body weight that is body fat. For example, if you weigh 150 pounds and have a body fat percentage of 10%, your body consists of 15 pounds fat and 135 pounds lean body mass.

Not all fat is bad. In fact, some body fats are essential to bodily functions. But how much is enough? Below you will find a chart that describes body-fat ranges in their associated categories. (Methods of measuring body-fat percentage can be found on the Fat Wars web site at www.fatwars.com, or you can go to www.fatwars.com and use the on-line body fat calculator.)

GENERAL BODY FAT PERCENTAGE CATEGORIES		
Classification	**Women (% fat)**	**Men (% fat)**
Essential Fat	10-12%	2-4%
Athletes	14-20%	6-13%
Healthy	21-24%	14-17%
Over-Fat	25-31%	18-25%
Obese	32% plus	25% plus

As you can see by the chart, a Healthy body fat percentage for a woman is between 21 and 24% and for a man between 14 and 17%. Unfortunately, the vast majority of North Americans are in the Over-Fat category and quickly inching their way toward Obese. I know this all too well, since I have personally tested the body mass of thousands of North Americans only to be greeted by a few people measuring within the Healthy status. I can almost count on one hand the individuals who tested within the Athletes range and did not classify themselves as athletes. You'll notice that athletes tend to have much lower body fat percentages. That's because they carry more muscle mass then the average person, which allows them to burn more fat.

OTHER WAYS TO MEASURE BODY FAT

Taking a body-fat percentage is the most accurate way to assess whether an individual is carrying an acceptable or excess amount of body fat. Still, the majority of health professionals use the Body Mass Index (BMI) as a way of assessing health risks associated with excess body fat. Your BMI is calculated with a formula that takes into account both weight and height. (In this case, size does matter!)

You can figure out your own BMI by using the easy-to-follow chart below, or the on-line calculator at www.fatwars.com. The ideal BMI is considered to be between 19 and 25. If your BMI is 25 or higher, you could be at risk for health problems associated with excess fat and obesity.

While the BMI is a useful guideline, it has some drawbacks: it places all weight (lean body tissue and body fat) in the same category; it doesn't differentiate between men and women; and it doesn't account for those folks (usually athletes) who have lots of muscle mass and are therefore heavier than average but are still in excellent shape.

Another important predictor of disease risk is your overall waist circumference, which is strongly associated with abdominal fat. A waist circumference of more than 40 inches in men and more than 35 inches in women signifies increased risk in those who have a BMI of 25 to 34.9.

Fat Wars Body Mass Index Chart

Height	Body Weight in Pounds																					
4'10"	91	96	100	105	110	115	119	124	129	134	138	143	148	153	158	162	167	172	177	181	186	191
4'11"	94	99	104	109	114	119	124	128	133	138	143	148	153	158	163	168	173	178	183	188	193	198
5'0"	97	102	107	112	118	123	128	133	138	143	148	153	158	163	168	174	179	184	189	194	199	204
5'1"	100	106	111	116	122	127	132	137	143	148	153	158	164	169	174	180	185	190	195	201	206	211
5'2"	104	109	115	120	126	131	136	142	147	153	158	164	169	174	186	185	191	196	202	207	213	218
5'3"	107	113	118	124	130	135	141	146	152	158	163	169	175	180	186	191	197	203	208	214	220	225
5'4"	110	116	122	128	134	140	145	151	157	163	169	174	180	186	192	197	204	209	215	221	227	232
5'5"	114	120	126	132	138	144	150	156	162	168	174	180	186	192	198	204	210	216	222	228	234	240
5'6"	118	124	130	136	142	148	155	161	167	173	179	186	192	198	204	210	216	223	229	235	241	247
5'7"	121	127	134	140	146	153	159	166	172	178	185	191	197	204	211	217	223	230	236	242	249	255
5'8"	125	131	138	144	151	158	164	171	177	184	190	197	203	210	216	223	230	236	243	249	256	262
5'9"	128	135	142	149	155	162	169	176	182	189	196	203	209	216	223	230	236	243	250	257	263	270
5'10"	132	139	146	153	160	167	174	181	188	195	202	207	215	222	229	236	243	250	257	264	271	278
5'11"	136	143	150	157	165	172	179	186	193	200	208	215	222	229	236	243	250	257	265	272	279	286
6'0"	140	147	154	162	169	177	184	191	199	206	213	221	228	235	242	250	258	265	272	279	287	294
6'1"	144	151	159	166	174	182	189	197	204	212	219	227	235	242	250	257	265	272	280	288	295	302
6'2"	148	155	163	171	179	186	194	202	210	218	225	233	241	249	256	264	272	280	287	295	303	311
6'3"	152	160	168	176	184	192	200	208	216	224	232	240	248	256	264	272	279	287	295	303	311	319
6'4"	156	164	172	180	189	197	205	213	221	230	238	246	254	263	271	279	287	295	304	312	320	328
BMI	19	20	21	22	23	24	25	26	27	28	29	30	31	32	33	34	35	36	37	38	39	40

Your Lean, Mean, Fat-Burning Machine

No government would dream of passing laws restricting your rights to eat whatever you choose. Can you imagine the outcry that would follow a ban on junk food? What this means is that if you want to win the Fat Wars, you're going to have to monitor your own food and lifestyle choices: you have to arm yourself with the right information and make decisions that will let your body become a lean, mean, *healthy* fat-burning machine. And the *Fat Wars Action Planner* is your ally in this transformation.

In *Fat Wars* you learned about the science of fat loss as oppose to weight loss. You learned how and why you store fat so easily, but most important you learned how to retrain your metabolism to mobilize and burn the fat you were living with. Now, you're ready to take the next step and put the principles you learned into a lifelong action plan. In the coming chapters you will embark on a new course of understanding your hormones and how the body works, and working with what nature designed. Along the way you'll learn how to speed up your metabolism, burn stored body fat, increase your ability to fight disease, create more energy, increase your life expectancy, and just plain look, feel, and perform better than you ever believed possible. Anyone who's tried to lose weight knows it's a tough battle. The *Fat Wars Action Planner* is designed to be your personal, long-term, workable lifestyle guide, focused on losing and keeping off *fat*, not *weight*.

So let's get started.

FAT WARS 101
Know Thy Enemy

Understanding the Enemy: The Skinny on Fat

Did you know that, of the 100 trillion cells that make up your body, only 30 billion of them—or 0.03%—are fat cells?

"Yeah, right," you might be thinking. "I've seen myself in the mirror. How could the fat that seems to form so much of my body actually make up such a small fraction of my cells?"

It's true: despite the amount of heartache they cause in terms of health problems and slights to body image, we have relatively few fat cells. Unfortunately, they're very wily, which is why they can wreak such havoc. Each and every one of these 30 billion tiny fat-manufacturing plants has the ability to expand up to a thousand times in volume. (They can shrink, too, but how often is that our problem?) To add insult to injury, they can also divide, creating more fat factories designed to beat us in the Fat Wars.

One important reason so many of us have lost so many battles with our fat cells is because we don't understand how they work. For example, we think we can starve them on low-calorie diets, only to become fatter than ever once the diet is over. Or, we try to cut out all carbohydrates, only to have the fat stick around after the inevitable carb binge.

One of the adages of war applies here: know thy enemy. Once you understand what makes your fat cells tick, you can arm yourself with strategies to outsmart them, and eventually win the battle against excess body fat. Eventually, you may come to see that fat cells were never designed to hurt you, but rather to save your life.

Our fat cells are so good at outsmarting us because they've been honing their strategies for millennia. Back in the days before agriculture, and well before the refrigerator and mini-mart, humans were hunter-gatherers who foraged for nuts and berries and enjoyed the occasional meal of wild game. It was a feast-or-famine world, and we survived by eating as much as we could when food was plentiful—and storing any extra calories in the form of fat. Because stored body fat was our only buffer during times of famine, our bodies eventually became very good (too good, you may be thinking) at converting almost anything we ate—excess dietary proteins and sugars, even extra hormones—into fat. And they became good fat hoarders, choosing in times of famine to sacrifice lean body tissue before fat stores.

Even though we've managed to eradicate the feast-famine cycle in much of the world, our bodies haven't changed their tactics, and they're not going to any time soon. As Drs. Mary and Dan Eades, the best-selling authors of *Protein Power*, put it, we're living with Fred Flintstone bodies in a George Jetson world. We've got to eat, drink, exercise, and live our lives to work in harmony with our caveman bodies.

In this and the following chapters, I will guide you on a reconnaissance mission designed to survey and gather information about your body and its strategies in the Fat Wars. Below, I'll discuss metabolism and thermogenesis, two biochemical processes key to how the body stores and burns fat. In Chapter 2, I'll discuss the hormone cycles that play such a huge role in the Fat Wars. With a little background knowledge, you can make your body's strategies work for you. And, in the process, you may well come to think of your body as an ally instead of an enemy.

Your Lean, Mean, Fat-burning Machine

You probably know someone who rarely exercises, eats like a horse, and never gains an ounce. (These people can be incredibly hard to like.)

Why have they managed to escape the Fat Wars—while others seemingly subsist on rice crackers and diet soda, go to aerobics class three times a week, and *still* seem to pack on the fat?

The answer, in part, lies in the efficiency of two body processes: metabolism and thermogenesis.

Metabolism

Your body is, essentially, an organic machine. It runs on millions of biochemical reactions that produce the energy we need to breathe, blink, sleep, think, and feel. Metabolism is the name for that series of reactions, which takes place in each of our 100 trillion cells.

Just like any other machine, the body needs fuel. It gets that fuel from food: carbohydrates, dietary fats, and dietary proteins, which it breaks down into the nutrients—vitamins, minerals, amino acids, and water—it needs to run. The quality and quantity of the fuel you provide your body will in large part determine how efficiently it runs, and whether it chooses to burn fat or store it. When the levels of various nutrients fall, the biochemical reactions fall right along with them, resulting in a slower metabolic rate—and excess body fat.

Once your body has digested the food you eat, it can do one of three things with the nutrients: use them immediately, store them within short-term energy reserves (that lie within your muscle and liver cells) called glycogen, or (and this is the kicker) store them within long-term energy reserves, called body fat. That's the option we'd like to avoid.

Of the energy that's used on the spot, approximately 80% is released as heat (through a process called thermogenesis, which I'll discuss below), while the rest does the other work of running your living systems. A fast, efficient metabolism can produce a lot of energy and heat (and consume a lot of fuel). In terms of winning the Fat Wars, then, we need to figure out how to devote the bulk of our nutrients to immediate energy or its short-term reserves, while training our metabolisms to avoid fat storage.

How do we do this? A few ways. First, because muscle is a prime site for fat burning, we want to build new muscle and/or maintain our current muscle stores at all cost. Second, we want to move those muscles through proper exercise (see Section III for a detailed discussion of exercise and an exercise action planner). Finally, we want to consume a higher-protein diet, which has been shown to boost metabolic activity through increased thermogenic activity (read on). A 1993 study by Dr. Barenys and his colleagues at Rovira University in Spain found that the combination of a higher-protein diet and moderate exercise increases the body's metabolic activity much more than a high-protein diet alone or exercise alone.

ATP: YOUR UNIVERSAL ENERGY SOURCE

Most people think that our digestive systems simply break down food and use it directly as energy. Well, it's not quite that simple. To get energy, our bodies must first convert the carbohydrates, dietary fats, and dietary proteins we eat into a universal energy substance, called adenosine triphosphate (ATP).

Each one of our cells has a tiny biochemical factory that can produce ATP, which is stored in muscle tissue. When the brain sends a signal along the nervous system to trigger a muscle contraction, enzymes break down ATP to release the energy required for the job.

All our energy starts with ATP. It's the required basic fuel for energy that doesn't require oxygen (short-term, anaerobic efforts) and for energy that does (longer-term, aerobic efforts). Although our bodies constantly make ATP, they also constantly use it up. That's because we use so much of it over the course of the day to move our muscles—from blinking our eyes and pumping our hearts to moving furniture. In fact, we use so much of it that the total amount required just to get most of us through a day would weigh in at an estimated 150 to 200 pounds!

Thermogenesis

Thermogenesis is just a fancy term for heat. If our metabolism acts as the generator for our systems by creating energy from fuel, then thermogenesis is akin to a furnace that creates heat in the body, keeping us at our ideal, constant body temperature of 98.6°F (37°C), even when we're sleeping. For this reason, thermogenesis is vital to life. And because it heats the body by burning excess calories from our stored fat supplies, thermogenesis is also a vital process in the Fat Wars.

Thermogenesis produces heat in three ways: through physical activity, by shivering to keep warm, and, oddly enough, by ingesting food. Every time you consume food, the body's core temperature rises slightly; in the process of releasing the nutrients from the food, a portion of that food's calories are "wasted" in the form of heat. What's interesting is that each macronutrient—that is, proteins, carbohydrates, and fats—has a different thermogenic value. In other words, different foods have varying heat-enhancing effects on the body, causing it to burn more or less fat.

Proteins have been shown to exert the greatest thermic value on the body. The thermic response from a high-protein meal can be 40% greater than that of a high-carbohydrate meal. For every 100 calories of protein eaten, for example, at least 20 calories are burned away as body heat (which mostly comes from fat)—compared to approximately 12 thermic calories for carbohydrates.

It's important to note that thermogenesis relies on body fat, and that it's therefore important to always have some body fat (a healthy body percentage) in storage. The more fat you carry on your frame, however, the less thermogenesis you create. That's because fat acts as a great insulator. It traps a great deal of heat inside the body; since less heat escapes, the body doesn't have to create more to keep itself warm. The opposite is true of lean people: with less fat to keep them warm, they must constantly generate heat—and burn fat. Thermogenesis, therefore, may just be one of the biggest reasons that thinner people can eat almost anything they want, whereas fatter people can gain fat almost by looking at food.

Thermogenic supplements: A hot topic!

Although you can increase thermogenesis naturally through diet and exercise, some natural supplements have been shown to enhance the body's ability to burn fat for heat. They include *ephedra* (or *Ma huang*), and *Citrus aurantium* (or *Zhi Shi*).

Both of these herbs stimulate fat burning by activating a specific group of cell receptors known beta-3 receptors, which increase the rate at which fat is released from both fat and muscle cells (lipolysis), and increase resting metabolic rate (thermogenesis), thus helping you to maintain or even build lean muscle mass while burning fat thermogenically.

These herbs have *also* been shown to reduce appetite, and to help stimulate active (brown adipose) fat cells to increase the oxidation of inert (white adipose) fat cells—which make up the excess fat you love to hate.

However, ephedra also activates other receptors that may cause blood-vessel constriction, a rise in blood pressure and possibly many other irregularities. Ephedra also happens to be an illegal substance in Canada.

Fortunately, *Citrus aurantium* (see Appendix) has been shown to raise metabolic rate *without affecting heart rate or blood pressure*. Preliminary research shows this herb induces a significant increase in metabolic rate, and that AdvantraZ™, a trademarked extract of *Citrus aurantium*, is an exceptional alternative to *Ma huang*.

Tea time!

Tea is one of the most widely consumed beverages in the world today, second only to water. But who would have thought that such a beloved beverage could offer hope in the Fat Wars Research performed at the University of Geneva and published in the *American Journal of Clinical Nutrition* in 1999 reported that green tea can increase the number of fat calories you burn by a whopping 35%.

The majority of the fat-burning effect is believed to be due to a class of compounds called polyphenols (substances that provide the plant with color) known as catechins (pronounced kat-a-kins) found in green tea—the strongest of which is referred to as epigallocatechin gallate (EGCG). When your body releases fat for energy, it releases a hormone called norepinephrine (see Your Body Chemistry Cheat Sheet pg. 85). The more norepinephrine, the greater the fat-burning effect. The problem is that norepinephrine has a limited lifespan in your body, meaning it only hangs around for a short time. This is where EGCG comes in. EGCG works to keep norepinephrine circulating longer—in turn helping your body burn more fat.

According to another study in the same journal in 2000, "Long term consumption of green tea may decrease the incidence of obesity and, perhaps, green tea components such as EGCG may be useful for treating obesity." All of these natural substances may be important arsenals in the Fat Wars. See the Appendix for Green tea recommendations.

2

HORMONES
Your Body's Greatest Ally

Invite a Caveman (or Woman!) to Dinner

We've all heard the saying, "You are what you eat." To a certain extent, it's true. When it comes to the Fat Wars, however, it may be more precise to say that we are what we *ate*—and I'm not talking about that double-bacon cheeseburger and chocolate milk shake you just had for lunch. I'm talking *way* back: I mean that humans are genetically programmed to function best on a diet similar to that of our distant biological ancestors: the prehuman hunter-gatherers who roamed the Earth more than 40,000 years ago.

Although we may look very different from those ancestors, we are in fact very similar to them genetically. According to Dr. Boyd Eaton, an expert in evolution and the diet of early humans, we share about 99% of the same genetic structure. What's more, roughly 99.9% of our genetic structure was formed before the advent of agriculture (10,000 or so years ago).

As I discussed in the last chapter, that structure was based on a cycle of feast and famine. The body that so stubbornly stores fat today was a survival mechanism for our ancestors, who never quite knew where or when their next meal would arrive. We're all here today because of that highly developed mechanism. Today, however, many of us are over-fat because our bodies haven't yet caught up to a twenty-first century in which famine, at least for most North Americans, is a phenomenon of the past.

The majority of us are no longer hunters, and gathering has been reduced to tossing economy-size bags of cookies and bagels into industrial-size shopping carts (and then tossing those bags into industrial-size cars that ensure we walk as little as possible). Dr. Eaton estimates that the early human diet was made up of at least 30% lean protein, along with unprocessed fruits, vegetables, nuts, and seeds. In contrast, according to research presented in the *Third National Health and Nutrition Examination Survey* from the U.S. Department of Health and Human Services, the average citizen in that country consumed a diet of 50% carbohydrates (most of them processed), 34% fats (and not the right kinds, as I'll discuss in Chapter 6), and only 15% protein (much of it not lean cuts, much of it highly processed). A 1996 national survey revealed that 88% of the U.S. population (90% of women and 87% of men) consume low-fat, reduced-fat, or fat-free foods and beverages. The largest numbers of fat replacers in these foods are carbohydrate-based.

If we invited the average prehuman over for a typical North American meal (spaghetti and meatballs with garlic bread, say), he or she would be completely bewildered by the food we eat. Small wonder then, that we're getting larger. We're giving our genes the wrong kind of fuel—kind of like low-octane gasoline for a high-powered race car. In the process, we're setting ourselves up for a range of diseases common to modern civilization but unheard of in prehistoric times: diabetes, cancer, heart disease, arthritis, autoimmune disorders … and obesity.

We're not going to win the Fat Wars by changing the way our genes function: geneticists estimate that it takes between 1,000 and 10,000 generations to substantially alter genetic makeup, and we don't have that kind of time. Since we're stuck with prehistoric bodies, we need to adopt a prehistoric way of eating, and that means eating a diet rich in lean protein, unprocessed carbohydrates, and, as I'll discuss in Chapter 6, the right kinds of fats.

The Generals of Your System

In theory, it makes sense: eat what you're genetically programmed to eat and your body will respond. But how does the theory work in practice? In other words: how does the body know what you're eating? How does it differentiate between protein and carbohydrates? Most important for your purposes, how does it decide whether you'll store or burn fat?

The answers lie in a group of regulatory substances in the body called hormones. Your body produces hormones in response to every-thing you eat, the amount and quality of your sleep, your exercise levels, how stressed you are—even the amount of sunlight you're exposed to or the lack thereof.

Not surprisingly, hormones play multiple, crucial roles in the Fat Wars. They act as messengers, relaying intelligence to the brain and various receptor sites in the body. They are gatekeepers: nothing gets by them as they allow or deny the body access to its stored fat as fuel. And they are generals, barking out commands to enzymes, who carry out their orders. Depending on the type of fuel, exercise, rest, and environment you give your body, you will stimulate your hormones to send either fat-burning or fat-storing messages to your cells.

The Fat Wars program is all about balance within this internal control system. It is designed to evoke a proper hormonal response that allows you to burn fat day and night. Powerful as they are, your hormones are under your direct control: you choose what food you'll eat and when, how and how often you'll exercise, and whether you'll expose yourself to undue stress or get proper rest.

In short, you want your hormones on your side in the Fat Wars. Treat them well, and they are your most powerful allies. Cross them, on the other hand, and they'll turn into a formidable enemy.

In this and the following chapters, I'll introduce (or reintroduce) you to the hormones that make or break you when it comes to the Fat Wars.

The Heavy Hitters: Insulin and Glucagon

We are what our ancestors ate. When it comes to the hormones insulin and glucagon, however, we're only as hormonally balanced as our last meal. These two hormones, both secreted from the pancreas, determine to a very large extent whether the body will store or burn fat.

Insulin

Prehistorically, insulin evolved to help us in times of famine by converting excess calories into storable forms of fat. It was our main fat-storage hormone, a role it still holds today—for better or for worse.

Insulin is secreted after we eat and following periods of elevated blood sugar. Under optimal conditions (the caveman diet), insulin is the body's friend. It deposits that blood sugar (glucose), along with amino acids (protein), in muscle so that we can move and function. It also synthesizes chemical proteins for building enzymes, hormones, and muscle. Insulin, however, is especially sensitive to dietary carbohydrates, which are metabolized quickly into sugar. And North Americans are carbohydrate junkies (remember the 50%).

Ask the average person, and he or she will likely tell you that carbohydrates are candies, bread, or pasta. That's true, but what most people don't realize is that fruits and vegetables are also carbohydrates. Believe it or not, you can gain unwanted pounds by consuming too many fruits and starchy vegetables. Carbohydrates are nothing more than various forms of simple sugars linked together in chains, which are broken apart during digestion. The faster a carbohydrate chain is broken, the faster its sugars are absorbed by the body. Carbohydrates can be classified according to the rate at which they break down in the body: the ones that give up their sugars quickest (usually highly processed white-flour and corn-based foods or junk foods) are "high-glycemic" carbs, while those that take longer to break down are referred to as "low glycemic" (more on this in Chapter 6).

The more carbs you ingest (especially the high-glycemic ones), the more insulin you secrete to clear the sugar from the bloodstream. When you consider that (if you're not diabetic) your entire bloodstream contains approximately 1 teaspoon (5 grams) of sugar at any one time, you may begin to get a sense of just how disruptive large amounts of dietary carbohydrates can be to your system. According to recent surveys, the average North American consumes almost 20 teaspoons (40 grams) of sugar every day.

So, what happens when there's excess insulin in the bloodstream? Quite simply, it's a victory for the dark side in the Fat Wars. High insulin levels stimulate the most powerful fat-storing enzyme in the body: lipoprotein lipase (LPL), which sets up your fat cells to store fat—and makes sure it stays stored (see Figure 2-1). The more high-glycemic, or insulin-stimulating, carbohydrates you consume, the more LPL your body secretes, and the fatter you become.

Although your body is designed to draw upon fat instead of sugar for 70% of its day-to-day energy needs, when insulin (and therefore LPL) levels are high, *they prevent the body from using its stored fat as fuel.* And so fat sticks around (you know where). In other words, too many of the wrong kinds of foods (high-glycemic carbs) can and will send a hormonal message, via insulin, to the fat cells. The message? "Time to store some fat."

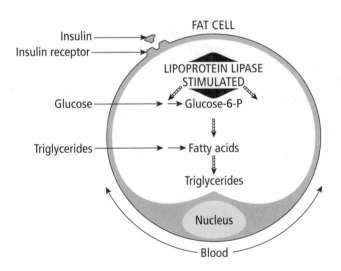

Figure 2-1: Too much insulin boosts fat storage by activating lipoprotein lipase.

Glycogen: Your Storage Tanks

Don't get me wrong: not all carbohydrates are bad. For optimum hormonal balance, we need to eat a certain amount of them each day. Carbs are the brain's primary energy source. The brain loves them— so much, in fact, that it uses at least two-thirds of the circulating sugars in the bloodstream while we are at rest. In order to ensure a continuous supply of high-octane brain fuel, the body must continual-ly convert dietary carbohydrates into available glucose.

The body, however, can use only a set amount of carbohydrates to generate immediate fuel. When it can't use sugars from dietary carbs immediately, the body stores them for future use in the form of long chains of glucose molecules called glycogen.

The body's glycogen containers are found in two areas: the liver and the muscles. The glycogen stored in the muscles is used as energy for the body but is virtually unavailable to the brain. Only the glycogen stored in the liver is accessible—through the bloodstream—as a backup source of brain food.

All this sounds well and good, and it is, until we consume too many carbs. That's because we have only a limited capacity to store glycogen. Even obese people can only store 300 to 400 grams of carbohydrate as muscle glycogen and another 60 to 90 grams in the liver. Anything more (with the handy help of insulin and LPL) finds its way to our fat cells. And if our liver and muscle glycogen tanks are always full (not a rare occurrence in a society where the average citizen consumes 156 pounds of sugar a year!), then approximately 70% of the sugar we ingest is stored immediately as body fat.

Understanding how insulin levels relate to increased fat gain will give you the knowledge to keep your 30 billion fat cells from growing exponentially. To free up the fat so that it can be burned in the muscle cells, you've got to lower your insulin levels. We can do that by exercis-ing properly and eating in harmony with our genetic structure—in other words, by eating like our prehistoric ancestors.

INSULIN, DIABETES, AND SYNDROME X

Say "insulin" and most of us tend to think of diabetes. There are many types of this disease, but the two most common forms are called Type I and Type II. Type I, which accounts for about 10% of cases, occurs when the pancreas malfunctions and does not secrete enough of the hormone insulin to lower blood-sugar levels. Type II diabetes (roughly 90% of cases), also called adult-onset dia-betes, occurs when insulin-receptor sites on the cells become insensitive to the hormone (usually after too much exposure to it). When this happens, insulin can't bind to the cells and release blood sugar into them, and both blood-sugar and blood-insulin levels remain elevated.

Over time, high levels of insulin and blood sugar can lead to an array of physiological changes, collectively known as Syndrome X and characterized by a cluster of interrelated symptoms that always includes insulin resistance.

Glucagon

Glucagon is the antagonist to insulin; when insulin levels are high, glucagon is low, and vice versa. Unlike insulin, glucagon is stimulated by protein (not carbohydrate) intake. And whereas insulin is responsible for preventing blood-sugar levels from climbing too high, glucagon ensures that they don't fall too low (like when we skip meals, exercise too much, or restrict calories too severely). Finally, whereas insulin (via lipoprotein lipase) sets us up for fat gain, glucagon, via a different enzyme called hormone-sensitive lipase (HSL), *sets us up for fat loss* by triggering the release of fat from fat cells (see Figure 2-2). Once liberated, the fat can be burned as fuel.

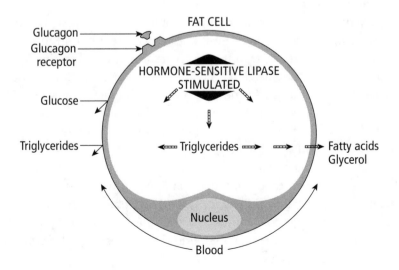

Figure 2-2: Glucagon stimulates hormone-sensitive lipase, which encourages fat burning.

HSL activity increases as glucagon is stimulated (through controlled carbohydrate and protein intake), while LPL activity increases when insulin is high, especially after a meal high in carbs and low in protein.

Stimulate glucagon and you'll burn fat. Sounds easy enough, doesn't it? Unfortunately (you were expecting this, weren't you?), there's a catch. If insulin and glucagon are present in the bloodstream in equal amounts, insulin will always win the tug-of-war between these two hormones. Fortunately, you can ensure that a tug-of-war never happens by changing the way you eat (as I'll discuss in Chapter 6).

As you will soon discover, the ratio of the macronutrients—protein, carbohydrate, and fat—in your diet can be more important to permanent fat loss then the overall calories you consume. Once you understand the ways in which foods control your biochemistry, you will be well on your way to victory in the Fat Wars.

THE THYROID GLAND: YOUR BODY'S THERMOSTAT

The endocrine hormones—T3, T4, and rT3—secreted by the thyroid gland play a key role in the Fat Wars. Remember the fat-burning processes of metabolism and thermogenesis? Well, the thyroid is like a thermostat, regulating the rate at which fat is burned and controlling the overall metabolic rate. A sluggish thyroid may therefore play a contributing role in obesity.

While rT3 (or reverse triiodothyronine) is the least active thyroid hormone, T3 (triiodothyronine) is the most active, and the one we want to stimulate most in the Fat Wars. Relatively inactive T4 (thyroxine) can be converted to T3 with the help of an enzyme (5-deiodinase) that cannot be formed without the mineral selenium. Since many North Americans are deficient in selenium, they may be missing out on the chance to increase their levels of active thyroid hormones—and burn more fat.

We can't blame all our fat woes on an underactive thyroid. It may well be, however, that many over-fat North Americans are suffering from a sluggish thyroid (hypothyroidism), characterized by symptoms that include cold hands and feet, high cholesterol and blood pressure, depression, constant fatigue, sleepiness, muscle weakness, brittle hair and fingernails, dry skin, constipation, and weight gain. If you think you may suffer from hypothyroidism, you can ask your doctor to test you for the condition. For an in-depth explanation of the workings of the thyroid, and information on how to self-test for hypothyroidism, please visit www.fatwars.com.

3

SMALLER FAT PEOPLE

Quick: How many diets have *you* been on?

Lost count? You're not alone. In fact, if you're like the bulk of North Americans, you probably stopped counting years ago. There's the annual I really will stick to it this time New Year's diet, the getting ready for summer diet, the pre-beach vacation diet, the I want my before-baby body back diet, the gotta look good for my high-school reunion diet ... you get the picture. As I mentioned in the introduction to this book, one-third of North American women and one-quarter of men are either starting or finishing a diet. We spend more than $33 billion annually on weight-loss products and services, skipping from one fad diet—low carbohydrates, no carbohydrates, high-protein, all-protein, low-calorie, low-fat, no-fat, no-fruit, grapefruit, you name it—to the next.

And you know what? None of them seems to work. In the short term, we may lose a few pounds, but over the long term only about 5% of dieters manage to keep off the lost weight. And the majority who don't are chagrined to find themselves fatter than they were *before* they started dieting. Obesity rates have tripled since our health experts warned us in the 1950s to lose weight by eating less fat and exercising more. In fact, despite all our diets, North Americans are getting fatter every year. And our doctors don't seem to have the answers.

When are we going to wake up and realize that the answer to obesity is more than caloric restriction and fat phobia? We're losing the battle of the bulge big time, and yet we won't admit it, perversely hoping against odds that the next diet will be the last one. Well, I can promise you one thing: if you continue a pattern of weight-loss attempts that involves the short-term pain of denying your body calories and nutrient groups, you are setting yourself up for failure. The best you can hope to achieve is becoming a smaller fat person. What do I mean by this? Read on.

Diets don't work because they fight our genetic makeup. They go against the way the body is designed to work—and remember, that design hails from prehistoric times. You may look like you're from the future, but the last time your body checked, you were still figuring out how to make the wheel. The body has been training for centuries on a feast/famine cycle. It knows well how to protect itself against the perceived famine of diets. It will win every time.

To truly lose fat (not simply weight)—and keep it off—you're going to have to forgo diets in favor of some lifelong lifestyle changes that incorporate exercise (especially muscle-building exercise) combined with a sustained balance of high-quality carbohydrates, dietary fats, and dietary proteins. You didn't get fat overnight, and you're not going to get, and stay, skinny over the course of a two-week fad diet. It doesn't sound glamorous or miraculous, and it will take real effort—but it's the only way to win the Fat Wars.

Muscle Matters

I've said it before, and I'll say it again: to win the Fat Wars, we have to maintain muscle at any cost. Muscle revs up our metabolism and increases thermogenesis, meaning we can burn more fat both while we're exercising and during rest. The more muscle we carry, the more fat we can burn for energy. And we're not talking piddly numbers here. Consider this:

- One pound of muscle can burn up to 50 calories a day.

- Fifty calories a day is 350 calories a week, or 18,200 calories a year.

- There are 3,500 calories in 1 pound of fat. Therefore every time you build a pound of new muscle, you gain the ability to burn 5 pounds of fat annually. And every time you lose a pound of muscle, you lose that ability.

Low-calorie diets are the enemy of muscle. That's because when the body is deprived of sufficient calories and nutrients, it begins to break down its own tissues to get energy (see Can Stress Make You Fat? below). That would be okay if it sacrificed excess fat, but it doesn't always work that way: the catabolic (breakdown) hormone cortisol attacks muscle big time, breaking it down into sugar to burn as energy.

At the end of a low-calorie diet, then, you're not really a thinner person: you're just a smaller fat person. To make matters worse, with all that muscle gone you now have a reduced capacity to burn fat. So you gain the weight back (plus a bit more), go on another diet, and the vicious cycle continues.

ARROWS DEPICT ENERGY RELEASE

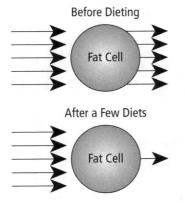

Figure 3-1: Dieting can prime your system for fat storage.

Can Stress Make You Fat?

Like just about everything else, we've also inherited our stress response from our prehistoric ancestors. In their case, stressful events usually meant physical threats—in the form of animal attacks, for example. They had two options: fight or flight.

Today, in our part of the world, we're less likely to be stressed out by physical threats. Instead, our stressors include things like illness, in-law visits, work, traffic jams, losing a job or a loved one, watching our teenagers come home with piercings, having too many bills to deal with—and going on calorie- and nutrient-restrictive diets. The hormonal response, however, is the same as if we were being cornered by a prehistoric beast.

When we're stressed, the body releases two specialized hormones from the adrenal glands: adrenaline and cortisol. These catabolic hormones give us the quick energy we (in theory) need to fight our stressor or retreat quickly. Cortisol breaks down sugars, dietary fats, and dietary proteins for immediate use. If there isn't a ready supply of new protein (amino acids) in the system, cortisol will take it from our body tissues in a process called gluconeogenesis—and muscle is the first tissue it plunders. It removes the nitrogen from the structural protein in our muscles and rapidly converts the amino acids to sugar for increased energy and maintenance of blood-sugar levels in the brain.

That's why stress (and cortisol) is a major enemy in the Fat Wars. It eats the muscle that we use to burn fat. This is a major reason we gain back weight after a diet—we've lost a key part of our fat-burning arsenal.

Chronic stress also works a number on our 30 billion fat cells. Researchers believe that stressing out may cause our fat cells to increase their fat-storing ability by cortisol stimulation of the fat-storing enzyme LPL (It appears that this chain reaction to fat storage from stress is greater in women than in men.). Excess stress also creates ravenous hunger signals within the brain. In nature, this signal prompts animals to replenish the energy reserves they squandered during the stressor.

So relax a bit: to win the Fat Wars, we've got to reduce cortisol levels, which means reducing stress. And when it comes to stress, perception equals reality.

Insatiable Cravings

Has this ever happened to you? You start yet another diet with the best intentions of sticking to it. And, for three days, you're good, dutifully eating only your prescribed skinless chicken breasts, celery sticks, and half-slices of bread. You ignore the ever-louder siren calls from the refrigerator—until the fourth day, when you succumb to your cravings. You order a pizza, and by the time it arrives, you've eaten half a jumbo tub of ice cream. After your carbohydrate fix is satisfied, you kick yourself for having no willpower. No wonder you can't lose any weight. And since you're depressed anyway, you finish off the ice cream.

Cravings are the downfall of so many failed dieters. You may be interested to know that cravings for carbohydrate-laden foods aren't simply a matter of willpower. They're actually part of a sophisticated hormonal and brain-chemical process set up to ensure that your brain is happy—even if you're not happy with the way you look in a bathing suit. Once you understand what's behind the powerful cravings you experience, you can take steps to minimize them.

The first bit of intelligence in the cravings puzzle is that carbohydrates—like cocaine—release morphine-like substances in your brain called beta-endorphins, which produce, literally, a high: a sense of well-being, increased self-esteem, and euphoria. That high is highly addictive, which is why we constantly crave more sugar once we've had even a bit.

Then the hormones and the brain chemicals kick in. Once we've come down from the initial beta-endorphin high, a sense of calmness and well-being sets in. That's the effect of the neurotransmitter (a chemical that relays messages from one brain cell to another) serotonin, also highly addictive.

Serotonin is our mood brain chemical. It plays a large role in sleep regulation, depression, anxiety, aggression, appetite, temperature regulation, pain sensation, and sexual behavior, to name a few. It's easy to see why the brain likes to keep optimum levels of the stuff circulating. Too little, and we may become depressed, moody, anxious, and unable to sleep. And the easiest way to keep serotonin levels elevated is to eat high-glycemic carbohydrates (aka junk food). The process goes something like this:

- The brain needs an amino acid, called tryptophan, to make serotonin. When other amino acids are in the bloodstream, however, tryptophan cannot get into the brain.

- When we eat carbohydrates, the body releases insulin to clear the sugar from the bloodstream.

- When insulin escorts glucose (the sugar) into the cells, it also escorts in the amino acids floating in the bloodstream—except for tryptophan. Thus, tryptophan has a chance to get into the brain uncontested.

- The brain can now produce serotonin, and we're happy again.

Unfortunately, it takes some time for serotonin to kick in after we begin eating carbohydrates, and so we keep right on eating until it does—easy enough when the high-fat, high-sugar foods taste so good.

If that weren't enough, nothing will cause insatiable cravings for sweet foods more than raising insulin by eating lots of processed foods. Lots of insulin in the bloodstream will bring down blood-sugar levels dramatically, causing hypoglycemic (excessive low blood sugar) episodes. These in turn trigger craving responses in order to quickly bring sugar levels up for the brain.

Galanin: An Unwelcome Guest

And here's the wrench in the works. As we keep plowing through the ice cream (or potato chips, or raw cookie dough), another neurotransmitter comes into play: galanin. (Cue the scary music.) This brain chemical is released once a certain amount of fat enters the body. Just as insulin competes with glucagon, galanin competes with serotonin—and quickly overpowers it, making us feel tired, passive, and confused. Oh, and it also creates a certain craving for fats.

Not surprisingly, galanin levels peak in the evening, which is why we can get through a day of successful dieting, only to succumb to cravings at night. Galanin is also triggered by reproductive hormones like estrogen (one of the reasons women who experience PMS crave fatty foods), stress hormones like cortisol, and our old friend insulin.

Just when you thought things couldn't get much worse, know this: galanin also plays a key role in making sure that extra dietary fat gets deposited directly into your fat cells.

How Can We Avoid Cravings, Then?

One way to keep serotonin levels up (without eating a half-dozen cinnamon rolls) is to maintain tryptophan levels naturally. It's important to consume enough low-glycemic carbohydrates to ensure that tryptophan is shuttled into the brain by insulin. We can also eat foods naturally high in tryptophan. They include milk, bananas, pineapple, chicken, turkey, soy, whey protein, and yogurt. High alpha whey protein happens to be one of the richest sources of tryptophan.

When we allow stress to overtake our lives, we massively deplete our serotonin tanks. Stress prompts the body to use tryptophan to manufacture not serotonin but other substances, such as vitamin B3 and NAD (the active coenzyme form of vitamin B3). A double-blind, placebo-controlled study published in the June 2000 edition of the *American Journal of Clinical Nutrition* indicated that whey protein containing high levels of alphalactalbumin could greatly increase plasma tryptophan levels in highly stressed individuals. High-alpha whey-protein powders, then, are not only another great source of tryptophan, but also provide a way to make sure it gets into the brain to manufacture serotonin.

A host of natural crave-free nutrients (see Appendix I) can help squelch excess cravings by eliminating nutrient deficiencies, balancing neurotransmitters, and lowering excess blood-sugar levels.

Deep restorative sleep is when serotonin and the other brain chemicals are restored for another day's work. Therefore, getting plenty of sleep is an important part of reducing cravings.

Finally, let's get back to the situation that got us craving in the first place: dieting. Low-calorie, low-carbohydrate diets—any diet that deprives us of nutrients—set us up to crave. So, in case I haven't yet made this clear: don't diet! In this book, I give you a range of strategies for eating well and exercising that will help you win the Fat Wars as part of a lifelong, workable, even pleasurable strategy. If you're not depriving yourself, you can help control cravings.

SCIENCE FINDS NEW KEYS TO UNDERSTANDING CRAVINGS

We know that it's next to impossible for most dieters to keep off lost weight for any substantial length of time. But gastric-bypass patients—who have had their stomachs drastically reduced via surgery—can lose hundreds of pounds and don't seem to gain them back. What makes the difference?

The answer may lie in a recently discovered hormone (found by Japanese researchers) called ghrelin, shown by British scientists in 2001 to trigger appetite in humans. In a study published in the prestigious *New England Journal of Medicine* in May of 2002, it was shown that dieting raises ghrelin levels—and, therefore, appetite—while gastric-bypass surgery sharply reduces them, to almost undetectable levels.

I'm not suggesting that you run out and sign up for gastric-bypass surgery! What these findings suggest, however, is that appetite is at least partially stimulated by a hormone. If scientists can discover an antagonist (or blocker) of ghrelin, they might be able to develop a safe way to help moderately over-fat people control their appetites.

And that's good, because a recent brain-imaging study at the U.S. Department of Energy's Brookhaven National Laboratory suggests that one reason obese people overeat may be that they find food more palatable than their leaner counterparts: the study found that the parts of the brain responsible for sensation in the mouth, lips, and tongue are more active in obese people than in normal-weight control subjects.

And, if you've ever thought of yourself as addicted to food, you may be right. The same researchers also found that obese people have fewer brain receptors for the neurotransmitter dopamine, which helps produce feelings of satisfaction and pleasure—from eating a good meal, for example. The study, published in the February 2001 edition of the medical journal *The Lancet*, suggests that obese people may eat more in order to stimulate their underserved reward circuits, just as addicts do by taking drugs.

A HORMONAL SOLUTION TO HUNGER PANGS

Looking for a natural way to reduce cravings and feelings of hunger? So are obesity researchers. And they're excited by a hormone called cholecystokinin (CCK), which can help control our hunger response.

CCK plays many essential roles in our gastrointestinal system. It stimulates the release of enzymes from the pancreas and increases gall bladder contraction and bowel motility. But it can also regulate our food intake by sending satiation signals to the brain, telling it that we're full. For this reason, it is a potential fat-loss aid. In animal studies, a rise in CCK is always followed by a large reduction in food intake.

Glycomacropeptides (GMPs) are low-molecular-weight protein peptides that exert an antibacterial and antimicrobial effect on our biochemistry. They are powerful stimulators of CCK. In human studies, whey-protein glycomacropeptides have been shown to increase CCK production by 415% within 20 minutes of ingestion.

Supplementing the diet with whey-protein isolates that contain GMPs, therefore, may help curb the appetite. But be careful when you're shopping: not all whey-protein isolates contain these important peptide fractions. Ion-exchange whey protein, for example, contains no or only trace amounts of GMP fractions. High alphalactalbumin whey protein, however, contains at least 20% of GMPs (see Appendix for whey protein with high alphalactalbumin levels).

So if you're looking for a natural way to reduce excess hunger pangs, look for higher-quality, cross-flow, microfiltered whey proteins that contain adequate amounts of GMPs. (And check the label!)

How Diets Don't Work: Your Diet Cheat Sheet

By now, it should be clear that dieting—that is, a short-term, all-or-nothing attempt to lose weight—is a losing effort (pun intended). Diets work against our genetic predisposition to store fat against famine; they trigger craving and fat-storing hormones while slowing down fat-burning ones, deplete us of fat-burning muscle, make us tired and cranky, and set us up to gain more fat once we return to our normal way of eating. Here's a quick glance at the three most common variations on the diet theme, and how and why they don't work.

DIET #1: BYE-BYE, CALORIES!	
How doesn't it work? You consume very little fuel, ensuring that you expend more calories than you take in. The math seems to make sense, doesn't it?	**What's the result?** • Sure, you'll lose some weight at the outset, but mostly in the form of water and precious, fat-burning muscle tissue (for every pound of fat you lose, you can also lose a pound of muscle), thereby reducing your metabolism. Since a lowered metabolic rate means that you can burn fewer calories, you'll gain weight more easily when you go off the diet. • Your body thinks a famine is on, triggering fat-storage enzymes like LPL. As soon as fuel consumption returns to levels close to normal, your cells will begin to hoard fat. • In response to a perceived famine, levels of a brain chemical called neuropeptide Y (NPY) increase, creating an insatiable appetite to which you eventually succumb. You go off the diet, often in a huge carbohydrate binge. • Because of your famine destroyed muscle tissue and lowered metabolic rate, you'll need even fewer calories than you did before. This ensures that even if you adjust to a new, reduced level of calories, you'll still pack on the fat.
DIET #2: BYE-BYE, FAT (AND HELLO CARBS)!	
How doesn't it work? You eliminate as much fat as you can from your diet, including essential fats. "I'm trying to lose fat," you think. "Isn't my best strategy not to eat any of it?"	**What's the result?** • Low-fat diets are generally disguises for high-carbohydrate diets. • We know that the body is very good at making fat from carbohydrates: by eating lots of carbs, you trigger insulin and LPL, your fat-storing enzyme. You're setting yourself up to store more fat.

- At the same time, you deprive your brain and body of essential nutrients that are found in fats causing you to have mood swings and possibly depression.
- Don't be fat-phobic!
- In fact, by avoiding the essential omega-3 fatty acids (especially preformed fish oils), you can actually increase your fat storage abilities.

DIET #3: BYE-BYE, CARBS (AND HELLO PROTEIN)!

How doesn't it work?
Since you know that carbohydrates make you fat, you cut them from your diet, replacing them with lots and lots of protein.

What's the result?

- You'll lose a few pounds at the beginning, but it will be mostly water. That's because one carbohydrate molecule can hold three or four water molecules.
- Don't forget that fruits and vegetables are also carbohydrates. By eliminating these valuable foods you are creating an acidic load on the body, thereby possibly setting yourself up for future bone loss and depriving your cells of life-giving phytonutrients.
- Because you don't have adequate carbohydrate levels to allow tryptophan to get to your brain, your serotonin levels will plunge.
- The body's way of getting the serotonin it needs is to crave sugary food to bring serotonin (and dopamine) levels up.
- The craving response will always override willpower. You'll go on an impossible-to-resist carb binge, and yet another diet will go down the tubes.

4

WAKING UP THINNER

We live in a go-go-go world whose motto seems to be, "The more sleep you get, the less productive you are!" Nothing, however, could be further from the truth. If you're one of those people who believes that getting enough sleep equals laziness, then you may be setting yourself up for failure in the Fat Wars. Proper sleep is essential to replenish energy reserves, rebuild and repair muscle tissue, reenergize the immune system, and cleanse the brain of excess cellular debris. More and more research points to the body's need for sufficient sleep in order to recuperate and burn fat effectively—and, by extension, to achieve fat-loss goals.

According to recent reports from the National Institutes of Health, Cornell University, and the Sansum Medical Research Institute at Santa Barbara, California (where insulin was first synthesized), to lose excess body fat, slow biological aging, and perform at peak energy efficiency, we need sufficient amounts of quality sleep. A 2002 study published in the *International Journal of Obesity* connected longer sleep duration with lower body-fat levels in 6,862 German children aged five to six years. The study showed that the prevalence of obesity (based on body-fat composition) in the subjects decreased as sleep duration increased, independent of other risk factors for childhood obesity.

The less sleep you get, the less likely you are to achieve your fat-loss goals. If that weren't enough, the fatter you are, the fewer calories you'll burn during sleep. You have a specific individual resting metabolic rate, or RMR, that dictates how many calories you'll burn within a twenty-four-hour period (and which is closely associated with your muscle mass and function). You also have a sleeping metabolic rate, or SMR, that dictates how many calories you burn during sleep. In another 2002 study, also published in the *International Journal of Obesity*, researchers measured the SMR in both obese and non-obese subjects. They found that the decline in metabolic rate during sleep is directly related to body weight—with the heaviest of the subjects having the lowest SMR.

You need enough sleep to ensure adequate production and secretion of two hormones that are incredibly important to the Fat Wars: melatonin and human growth hormone (HGH). I discuss these below.

Sleeping on Hormonal Schedule

Since we have virtually the same genetic structures as our prehistoric ancestors, the same internal clock that governed them also governs us. That clock is located in the center of the brain and is comprised of two tiny neural structures, called the suprachiasmatic nuclei (don't even try to pronounce this one). All bodily processes revolve around the intricate timing of this biological clock, which is still controlled by light and dark. In other words, our bodies were designed to function—and still do—around the rhythms of sunrise and sunset, what researchers refer to as the circadian rhythms of nature.

Our biological clocks regulate the natural rhythms of wakefulness, body temperature and, most important, the timing of hormone production over the course of each twenty-four-hour cycle. Specific hormones are produced at specific times of the day and night—or, at least, they should be.

Specialized sex hormones, for instance, are naturally high in the morning, as are stress hormones like noradrenaline (brain adrenaline) and cortisol. Specific neuropeptides (brain chemicals), such as dopamine, also rise in the morning to increase alertness and stimulate us into a "gotta have it" mode of action. In prehistoric times, morning would be the time to mate, hunt, and gather our daily supplies before the nightfall. Today, it might mean that we do our best thinking, exercising, negotiating, and work (not to mention lovemaking!) in the morning.

In the evening, sex and stress hormones (especially cortisol) fall. The rose light of the setting sun automatically blocks the green spectrum of daylight at what's known as the preoptic site in your brain, stimulating the release of your sleep hormone, melatonin, the most powerful antioxidant known to science.

Melatonin lowers your body temperature (one of the reasons you need a blanket to sleep—even in the summer), which in turn lowers your sex hormone and cortisol levels. It takes approximately three and a half hours of straight melatonin production to produce one of your strongest immune regulatory agents—prolactin. Prolactin was once thought to be necessary only for lactation in mammals, but research has now confirmed its necessity in enhancing the immune system's T cells and NK (natural killer) cells—our first lines of defense against cancer.

Melatonin is also essential for preserving brain tissue. Your brain is almost 60% fat, most of which is polyunsaturated fat (the good stuff). This makes it highly susceptible to free radical attack and destruction. (Free radicals are unstable molecules that can damage cell structure and lead to disease.) The most destructive free radical produced in your body is the hydroxyl radical, which is so powerful it can actually destroy your cellular blueprint—DNA. Melatonin happens to be the most effective substance in stopping the hydroxyl radical in its tracks.

When it comes to melatonin—and creating the best environment for brain integrity and optimum health—timing is everything. Melatonin cannot be produced during daylight hours or, for that matter, in the presence of artificial (non-sunlight) light! For optimum melatonin synthesis, the darker the environment the better. This means sleeping without any lights on (including night-lights, the light from the clock radio, the television, and so on). Need proof of this? What about the fact that animals in nature—who aren't exposed to artificial light—rarely, if ever, get cancer? Only domesticated animals, raised under electric light, succumb to this devastating disease.

Research has shown that the average body needs approximately six hours of straight prolactin production to modulate immunity. Since prolactin is secreted only after three and a half hours of melatonin production, you may need up to nine and a half hours of sleep each night to create an optimum environment for your body's defense force.

When we allow ourselves to fall out of sync with nature's clock by staying up late into the evening or missing valuable sleep, our hormonal rhythms begin to run amok. When our bodies can no longer produce enough of the hormones they need at the right time—or when hormonal messages are not heard as loudly as they once were—our bodies begin to experience a decline in function. As T.S. Wiley and Bent Formby, Ph.D, two researchers from the Sansum Medical Research Institute, suggest in their book *Lights Out*, "sleep is the best immunological defense mechanism you could ever wish for."

TO NAP OR NOT TO NAP?

According to Cornell University sleep researcher Dr. James Mass, naps are a great idea—but only if you are unable to get one continuous period of sufficient nighttime sleep that leaves you feeling alert throughout the day.

Any nap longer than 30 minutes, however, can contribute to problematic nighttime insomnia. After 30 minutes of continual sleep, your body shifts into delta, or deep, sleep. It's difficult to wake from the delta state, and when forced out of it—by an alarm clock, for example—you will probably be disoriented and groggy. For optimal rest, then, nap only for between 15 and 30 minutes. If you are severely sleep deprived and need longer than 30 minutes to feel fully rested, then sleep specialists recommend napping for an hour and a half to complete a full sleep cycle.

HGH: Your Greatest Fat-Burning Ally

If sleep is your greatest asset when it comes to rebuilding, repairing, and replacing your worn-out, damaged cells, then human growth hormone—adequate levels of which depend on deep sleep—is one of your greatest fat-burning allies. During sleep, you switch from a catabolic (breakdown) state to an anabolic (rebuild) one. HGH, produced in the pituitary gland within the brain, controls much of this anabolic state.

One of HGH's main jobs is to regulate growth, especially at puberty. HGH has also been called the ultimate antiaging therapy. It affects almost every cell in the body, rejuvenating the skin and bones; regenerating the heart, liver, lungs, and kidneys; and bringing organ and tissue function back to youthful levels. HGH revitalizes the immune system, lowers the risk factors for heart attack and stroke, improves oxygen uptake, and helps to prevent osteoporosis.

In terms of the Fat Wars, HGH is also responsible for increasing lean body mass (muscle) and decreasing stored body fat by freeing it up as an energy source. It is secreted in rhythmic pulses from the pituitary gland throughout the day and night, but primarily while you sleep. In fact, up to 80% of HGH is produced while you are in your deepest phase of sleep (as long as enough melatonin is secreted). HGH hangs around in the bloodstream only for a few minutes, but don't let its fleeting appearance deceive you. It is a very powerful weapon in the war against body fat. In these few minutes, it makes its way to your 30 billion fat cells, where it latches onto specific growth-hormone receptors, activating the release of stored fat for energy. Perfect.

As you can see, HGH is powerful stuff. In fact, in one of the most famous studies to date, led by the late endocrinologist Dr. Daniel Rudman, HGH was able to reverse the loss of muscle mass and the gain in body fat in elderly men. At the end of this study—presented in the *New England Journal of Medicine* in 1990—those who received HGH gained an average of 8.8% muscle and lost 14% fat (and the youngest man was sixty-one years of age).

When released, HGH also goes to the liver, where it stimulates the release of a set of hormones known as insulin-like growth factors (IGF), also known as somatomedins. As their name suggests, they bear a strong structural resemblance to insulin, and are required for growth of cells, bones, muscles, organs, and the immune system.

In Chapter 6, you'll learn more about the three basic sources of energy the human body relies on: carbohydrates, dietary fats, and dietary proteins. Carbohydrates must be converted into glucose before the body can use them as an energy source. As you have learned, excess glucose is converted into glycogen and stored, although the body only has a limited storage capacity within its glycogen tanks. Once a good supply of the glycogen has been used up, the body enters a semi-fasting mode and begins burning fat. HGH is responsible for switching it into this fat-burning mode.

Destroying Your Nighttime HGH Levels

By now, it should be clear that HGH is a key part of our arsenal against not only excess fat, but ill health. Therefore, it's important to ensure optimum conditions for its manufacture.

Unfortunately, time is against us in this pursuit. After our early twenties, HGH declines approximately 14% per decade; around the age of sixty we have experienced an 80% decline in the hormone. IGF levels follow closely behind, with a decline of nearly 50% soon after middle age (forty). It is widely believed that these prodigious hormonal declines are directly responsible for robbing us of our youth, and for the midlife bodily transformations that we have all come to fear.

Remember: up to 80% of HGH is produced during sleep. Many obese individuals, however, have difficulty sleeping because of a condition called obstructive sleep apnea (OSA), which makes it difficult to stay asleep long enough to fall into the deeper sleep cycles where HGH is secreted. As a result, their HGH production becomes incapacitated. Studies show that OSA affects more than half the obese population. Neck circumference in men and BMI in women seem to be the strongest predictors of the severity of this condition in obese patients. Morbid obesity can often be associated with excessive daytime sleepiness, even in the absence of sleep apnea.

Diet and insulin levels also affect the production and release of HGH. If you, like most North Americans, maintain high insulin levels throughout the day and evening by consuming lots of high-glycemic carbohydrates, then your HGH levels could be low. Numerous studies reveal that high insulin levels negatively affect our body's anabolic (rebuild and repair) response by lowering HGH production.

To achieve optimal, natural HGH secretions, then, we need to go to bed early and achieve sound sleep from 11 p.m. to 2 a.m. We need to adjust the way we eat so that insulin levels are not elevated. (I can't stress that enough). Getting regular, strenuous exercise and remaining free of disease are also important ways to ensure adequate HGH levels.

NATURE'S WAY TO HIGHER HGH LEVELS

Nearly half the pituitary gland, where HGH is produced, is comprised of growth hormone-producing cells (called somatotrophes). Amazingly, these cells can be stimulated to produce youthful amounts of HGH at any age. In 1995, Dr. William Sonntag and his colleagues at the Bowman Gray School of Medicine in North Carolina completed a study showing that the age-related decline in HGH secretion is reversible—naturally. That's great, given the fact that two-thirds of our population will lose one-third of their muscle by the time they are sixty and gain the rest of their body mass in excess body fat. We can use all the natural help we can get!

Bioavailable growth factors occur naturally in high concentrations in life's first food, colostrum (the first secretion of mother's milk after birth). Fortunately, bovine colostrum (from cows) can be found on your local health-food-store shelves. But if you decide to use this natural food, make sure it is extracted—using low heat—from the first milking (within the first six hours) of Grade A dairies (see Appendix for recommendations).

Many companies have designed or are designing HGH-secreting agents called growth hormone stimulators (or potentiators). One class of these stimulators is referred to as "secretagogues." A secretagogue is a substance, chemical, or nutrient that helps stimulate a gland to release a hormone. Some of the best and safest secretagogues available are comprised of various mixtures of amino acids, including glutamine, arginine, lysine, ornithine, tryptophan, leucine, and glycine. These natural substances, if used under proper guidance, may presently be one of the safest and best ways to achieve higher HGH levels in the body. (See Appendix for recommendations.)

Whichever way you decide to increase your HGH levels, I advise staying away from any products that contain actual HGH unless directed otherwise by your physician.

5

HIS AND HERS DESIGNER FAT CELLS

Why is it that men don't seem to gain fat as easily as women? And how come when a man and a woman go on the same diet, he loses more weight, faster (even when he cheats a bit, the dog)? If you've ever wondered why men and women seem to be fighting different battles in the Fat Wars, look no further than the metabolic advantage extra muscle offers, and at the hormones estrogen and testosterone, which dictate to a large extent how much muscle you presently have. While these so-called sex hormones in large part regulate sexual and reproductive function, they also have many other roles. And, perhaps not surprisingly, they play a key part in the Fat Wars.

Given that men and women have different genetic programs (women are designed to ensure the survival of offspring, which dictates, among other things, that they will have a much larger body-fat percentage than men), it makes sense, at least evolutionarily, that male and female bodies take different approaches to the manufacture, use, and storage of fat. This means that men and women will have to take slightly different approaches when it comes to stimulating the body to burn fat—especially as they age.

His Fat

Testosterone is the most important of the male hormones collectively called androgens. And it's a big deal in the Fat Wars. When naturally abundant (as it is in most healthy young men—those ripped guys on the beach who chow down on subs and beer and don't seem to gain an ounce), it is the core of men's energy, stamina, and sexuality. It's also what keeps them lean. Testosterone helps build muscle (a key fat burner) and bone and improves oxygen uptake throughout the body (important for thermogenesis, or burning body fat). Testosterone also helps control blood sugar, which means that it helps minimize insulin levels—and therefore fat manufacture and storage.

Testosterone and obesity have a direct, inverse relationship. As testosterone levels increase, obesity decreases, and vice versa. A 1998 study of 284 middle-aged men, for example, conducted by Swedish researchers, showed that low testosterone levels were both directly and indirectly related to the amount of fat men carried around their midsections. An adult male's testicles normally produce between 7 and 10 milligrams of testosterone per day; in over-fat or obese men, that amount declines in direct proportion to the degree of obesity.

Unfortunately, testosterone levels also decline with age, a gradual process that begins after about the age of thirty-five. That's when men start noticing a gradual loss of muscle mass. Since muscle is so important when it comes to fat burning, losing any of it paves the way to the accumulation of fat—which is why aging men also start to get fatter.

Not all testosterone is created equal. Free, biologically active (or "unbound") testosterone and testosterone bound to albumin are the forms of the hormone that do most of the work in the body. Inactive testosterone, on the other hand, is bound to a specific protein known as sex-hormone-binding globulin (SHBG), and is therefore prevented from doing much. Unfortunately, it's the active form of testosterone that declines as men age.

Help Is on the Way

Amazingly, many of the signs of aging associated with decreased testosterone can be reversed when the hormone is restored to optimal levels. Brain function improves, as do cardiovascular function, bone strength, and—most important—muscle mass, which sets the stage for a decrease in body fat.

So, how do men get back some of their lost testosterone?

In a few ways. Exercise is one—but not any old exercise. While many people think that aerobic activity is the best way to go, in fact only weight-resistant exercise has been shown to raise testosterone levels effectively. (Don't avoid aerobic exercise completely, though: when weight training and aerobic activity are combined, the benefits of both are enhanced. See Section III). A second way to increase testosterone levels is to unbind the testosterone bound to SHBG, thus freeing it up to do its good works in the body. Extracts of stinging nettle root (*urtica dioica*), a natural substance, has been shown to help release testosterone from SHBG (and to help prevent and perhaps even treat prostate disease). Special compounds in the plant known as lignans have a high affinity to SHBG; they bind to the hormone, in the process setting free the testosterone. (If you're considering trying a stinging-nettle supplement, look for products that have been extracted using water or methanol; those with alcohol or ethanol extracts aren't nearly as effective, or are not effective at all—see Appendix for recommendations.)

Another natural extract that shows great promise in boosting testosterone is elk velvet antler, or EVA. This extract, which comes from elks' antlers, has long been in use in Asia but has only recently garnered attention in the West as a rich source of biological substances that include growth hormones, amino acids, and natural anti-inflammatory agents. Most interesting for this discussion is the fact that EVA, taken orally, was shown in a 1998 University of Alberta study to significantly boost human testosterone levels.

Ensuring adequate protein intake (a recurring theme in the Fat Wars) is another way to help boost testosterone levels by lowering SHBG. A study published in the January 2000 edition of the *Journal of Clinical Endocrinology and Metabolism* showed that elderly men with low dietary protein intakes had elevated SHBG levels and lower amounts of active testosterone.

The mineral zinc is another powerful friend of testosterone. Not only is zinc an integral part of the enzymatic pathways that manufacture testosterone, but it also has the ability to inhibit the production of a powerful metabolite of testosterone called dihydrotestosterone (DHT). DHT has been blamed for years by urologists for benign prostate enlargement and has also been deemed a major culprit in hair loss on the top of the head.

An Unwelcome Transformation!

As a man ages, depleted and/or bound testosterone is far from the only problem he faces. As men experience a drop in their testosterone levels (or a rise in their SHBG levels), they usually experience a rise in their estrogen levels, too. Say what? It's bad enough that as men age they lose their main metabolic engines (muscle) all the while gaining extra fat, but biology has yet another cruel trick up its sleeve. As men's fat cells start to increase in size, the fat cells start to manufacture a special enzyme called aromatase. Aromatase lives in fat, and the more body fat we produce, the more of this enzyme gets made. Aromatase is responsible for converting what is left of our valuable testosterone production to estrogen. And as we are producing more and more estrogen, we are losing more and more muscle and gaining more and more fat. In fact it's not uncommon for a man of retirement age to have a higher estrogen content in his body than a woman of the same age, as long as she is not on estrogen replacement therapy. Yikes!

More Help

In addition to inhibiting SHBG binding, stinging nettle root has also been shown to help inhibit testosterone-conversion activity. But one of the most powerful conversion inhibitors to date is a bioflavonoid called chrysin. Chrysin was shown to be similar in both potency and effectiveness to the conversion-inhibiting drug aminoglutethimide. For chrysin to become bioavailable to the body, it must be accompanied by an enhanced delivery ingredient, such as piperine (black pepper extract). See the Appendix for product recommendations.

LOSING IT THROUGH STRESS

Allowing yourself to excessively stress out over life's ups and downs is one way of guaranteeing testosterone goes out the window. Stress has been shown to create a dramatic drop in testosterone levels. A man's testosterone levels can drop by as much as 50% in times of stress. Bottom line, get a grip on your perception of reality.

Newer Options in Testosterone Replacement

When it comes to artificial testosterone replacement, North American men are benefiting from the recent release of some safe, efficient products that have been successfully used for many years in Europe. In addition to synthetic testosterone injections and oral forms of the hormone (which are not necessarily exactly the same as the testosterone men create naturally), men can now use natural testosterone patches or creams that are rubbed into the skin.

I recommend that men looking to replace testosterone opt for a natural, bio-identical product. These products, synthesized in laboratories as exact molecular duplicates of the stuff our bodies produce naturally, seem to present no apparent health risks when taken under the care of a qualified physician. They are available, with a prescription, through compounding pharmacies or by mail order, and include Testoderm (a patch), Androderm, and AdroGel (1%), a new dihydroxytestosterone gel.

Her Fat

I'm going to come right out and say it: women lack men's arsenal when it comes to winning the Fat Wars. Let's look at the facts. Because of the evolutionary impulse to bear and nurture offspring, women's fat cells are up to five times larger than men's, contain up to twice the fat-storing enzymes, and can contain half the fat-releasing enzymes. Women also have at least 8% more fat (that's an extra 120,000 calories in storage!) than their male counterparts, and, on average, about 40 pounds less of fat-burning muscle. As well, women have a tenth of men's levels of testosterone (yes, women's bodies contain testosterone, just as men's contain some estrogen), and we know that testosterone is a muscle-building, fat-burning hormone. Due to the extra muscle mass, men can burn up to 30% more calories than women—during exercise and at rest.

BECOMING MUSCLE-BOUND?

Testosterone happens to be one of the most important hormones when it comes to the body's fat-burning ability, because humans can't build an ounce of muscle without it. Estrogen, on the other hand, is a pro-fat hormone that encourages the deposits of extra fat around a woman's hips, breasts, thighs, and buttocks. Estrogen-affected fat cells tend to hold on to fat more stringently, and to release it more grudgingly than cells not influenced by estrogen. This is why women should never be concerned with becoming muscle-bound or putting muscle on too easily. Along with proper weight training, muscle development requires the message of testosterone in order to become part of one's structure, and since women have a limited supply of the hormone to start with, they can use all the help they can get.

Vive la difference! It may not be fair, but it's true, and it relates in large part to estrogen.

Estrogen is actually a combination of three different hormones: estriol, estradiol, and estrone. It is produced in the ovaries (and to a lesser extent in the adrenal glands). Together, these hormones perform more than three hundred functions in the body, from building bones and strengthening the heart to regulating the brain. Estrogen is important stuff.

Like testosterone in men, estrogen production in women begins to decline in the mid-thirties (a period known as perimenopause). And because the hormone is so important, the female body begins to devise ways to keep estrogen levels up. Since the ovaries and adrenal glands are slowing down their production, women's bodies turn to fat to take up the slack. That's right: fat, under the right circumstances, can become an estrogen factory.

Once estrogen levels get below a certain point, the female body comes up with a host of ways to pump up fat stores. It steps up fat-storing enzymes and slows down production of fat-releasing enzymes to make sure it has plenty of fat to work with. Just in case, fat cells can also split during this time. As well, as I discussed in Chapter 3, a drop in serotonin levels as women age causes them to crave carbohydrates, which, when ingested in excess, ensure even more fat production.

To add insult to injury, women's bodies protect and add to their new fat stores by doing away with fat-burning muscle. Unless she takes steps to preserve it, a woman typically loses half a pound of muscle each year during perimenopause, replaced by a full pound and a half of fat! That may not seem like much, but over twenty years, it means that the average woman gains 30 pounds of pure fat.

All that new fat seems to gather predominantly in one spot: the tummy. Know why? Because the fat in this area—which insulates the adrenal glands and liver—is most conducive to producing estrogen. The adrenal glands produce a type of testosterone, and the liver produces an enzyme that converts that testosterone to estrogen within the manufacturing plants of the fat cells.

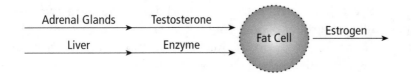

Figure 5-1:
The estrogen production line

Can't We have It Both Ways?

All in all, the female body has done an effective job of protecting its estrogen stores. And it has good reason to: the estrogen produced in the fat cells is designed to play an important role in menopause. It reduces hot flashes to half of what thinner women experience, allows for better sleep and healthier skin, and, most important, cuts osteoporosis risk (again to half the levels that thinner women experience).

The challenge, then, is this: is it possible to reap the benefits of estrogen without having to pack on weight?

The answer, fortunately, is yes. Of course, diet and exercise play a vital role in the Fat Wars. By combining a higher-protein, lower-carbohydrate diet with weight-training exercise, women have taken the first steps toward preserving valuable muscle and keeping fat in check. But beyond these steps, women have at least a couple of strategies at their disposal to combat the body's efforts to hoard fat as it ages.

Estrogen-replacement therapy (ERT)

The first strategy to deal with declining estrogen is to replace it. And women do in droves: at 50 million prescriptions a year, ERT in its various forms is the most widely prescribed drug in North America.

But what are women getting with synthetic drugs? Generally, a form of estrogen that is much stronger and very little like the combination of hormones their bodies originally produced. The most common form of ERT, Premarin, is in fact synthesized from pregnant mares' urine (hence the name).

While many women do fine on synthetic ERT, many others tolerate these foreign forms of estrogen less well. Either way, I personally believe that if women choose ERT, it is important to supplement the human body with natural hormones that are identical to the ones our bodies synthesize. If you are taking synthetic ERT, or are considering taking it, I strongly urge you to consult your physician about alternative sources of natural estrogens—Bi-Estrogen and Tri-Estrogen are two—that compounding pharmacies can supply. Also ask your doctor about prescribing natural progesterone, a precursor hormone that converts into other hormones in the body, including estrogen and testosterone, and as such, should generally be taken along with estrogen.

Soy good for you!

The second strategy to deal with declining estrogen takes a different approach: it mimics the effects of estrogen in the body so that the body is fooled into thinking it has all it wants of its precious hormone. As a result, the female body doesn't feel the need to aggressively pack on the fat.

Phytoestrogens are plant compounds that contain estrogen-like molecules, which are able to bind to the same receptor sites in the body normally occupied by the body's own estrogen. They also emit weak estrogen-like signals to the body. And they ease lots of symptoms of menopause: they reduce the severity of hot flashes, irritability, mood swings, and anxiety. They can help lower bad cholesterol—LDLs—thus lowering risk of heart disease, and, in some cases, they may lower the risk of osteoporosis and breast cancer. Our main interest here, however, is in phytoestrogens' ability to help us lose fat—or not gain it in the first place.

Where do we get phytoestrogens? More than three hundred plants are known to contain them, but the most common source for them is soy products. Fermented soy products, like firm tofu, miso, or tempeh, however, are the most valuable sources. The traditional Japanese process of fermentation helps preserve a class of compounds in soy products called isoflavones, wherein soy's magic seems to lie. Soy contains many isoflavones, but genestein, diadzein, and glycitin have been most thoroughly researched and are responsible for the food's powers. All this news on soy doesn't mean that you should make it the staple of your diet. Too much soy may not necessarily be the best thing. As I mentioned, soy does exert a slight estrogenic effect on the body, and any excess estrogen (phyto or the real deal) can have a counter-effect in your body's war against fat. In my opinion, soy is good only in moderation.

Some soy researchers have even cautioned women on using excess amounts of soy products due to their possible suppression of thyroid function. Dr. Michael Fitzpatrick, one of these researchers, has pointed out that as little as 30 milligrams of soy isoflavones (the amount in 5 to 8 ounces of soy milk) have been proven to suppress thyroid function. Larrian Gillespie, M.D., recommends persons with lazy thyroid avoid soy altogether.

SOY IN A SHAKE

In addition to fermented soy foods, soy-based protein shakes are a good way to get a quick hit of phytoestrogens and isoflavones. For this reason, and because they're an easy way to add high-quality protein to the diet, I highly recommend protein shakes as part of your Fat Wars arsenal. But when you shop for a protein powder, please be aware that they're not all created equal. Many soy proteins (as well as many soy products) are poorly produced, using an alcohol extraction method that removes most, if not all, of the active isoflavones. Choose only water-extracted soy protein and fermented soy-protein isolates: they will retain their natural isoflavone advantage. If you can, try to mix soy protein with high-quality whey-protein isolate (more on this in the next chapter) or look for combinations of these two already mixed (see Appendix for recommendations).

> Also keep in mind that the majority (57%) of soy products cur-
> rently on the market come from genetically modified (GMO) soy. If
> you're at all concerned about GMO foods—and I am—choose soy
> products marked non-GMO. Better yet, choose certified organic soy
> products.

Eat your veggies to alter estrogen metabolism

Numerous middle-aged women and men suffer needlessly from a condition referred to as estrogen dominance, in which healthful estrogens
are pushed out of the way by unhealthful estrogens. That's right, there
are good estrogens and bad estrogens. The bad ones—referred to as 16-
hydroxy estrone and estradiol—promote more active fat storage and
larger fat cells. The good ones—referred to as the 2-hydroxy estrogens—support the mobilization of stored fat, making exercise and nutrition that much more efficient at reducing fat stores.

New research confirms that hormone metabolism changes with age.
As Michael A. Zeligs, MD, a physician and nutritional expert from Boul-
der, Colorado, puts it, "Slower hormone metabolism in midlife can
mean higher than normal levels of estrogen and a deficiency in its beneficial 2-hydroxy metabolites." It is these 2-hydroxy metabolites, deemed
the good estrogens, that are able to support needed progesterone production in middle-aged women, protect against certain forms of cancer
(especially breast and uterine), and help mobilize stored fat in both
women and men. The overproduction of bad estrogens (the 16-hydroxy
variety) directly contributes to obesity.

Myriad research confirms that extracts from the indole family found
only in cruciferous vegetables—cabbage, broccoli, bok choy, Brussels
sprouts, cauliflower, kale, kohlrabi, rutabaga, and turnip—may provide
the answer to some of these estrogen-related problems. Two such miracle extracts are indole-3-carbinol (I3C) and diindolylmethane (DIM).
In numerous studies, both I3C and DIM have positively influenced the
way estrogen is metabolized, favoring the good estrogens—2-hydroxy
metabolites—instead of bad ones—16-hydroxy estrogens.

And Baby Makes Three

By now, it's no secret that advancing age can be a key disadvantage in the Fat Wars. As we grow older, the hormones that help keep us lean decline, while those that send fat-storing messages merrily proliferate. The older we get, the harder we have to work at keeping fat in check.

How, then, do we account for the (literally) ballooning statistics for obesity in North American kids? Nearly one-third of our children are over-fat. One in five is considered obese. Obese teens have a greater than 50% chance of becoming obese adults—odds that climb to 80% if they have an obese parent.

And this isn't just cute baby fat: being over-fat or obese places children and teens at a higher risk for the same ugly health conditions as over-fat adults. (And let's not forget the depression and low self-esteem that can go along with being over-fat; kids can be cruel.) Perhaps the most notable symptom of a new trend toward childhood and teen obesity is the epidemic of Type II diabetes, which until recently was known as adult-onset diabetes. It's hardly surprising in a world where our kids down liquid sugar in the form of soda pop at unprecedented rates, and feed on diets rich in highly processed, sugary, carbohydrate-heavy convenience and fast foods. Today's kids are less physically active than kids of earlier generations, another factor that contributes to the epidemic.

If you're the parent of an over-fat or obese child, or if you're fighting the Fat Wars yourself and want to ensure that your offspring stay lean, remember that healthy eating and adequate exercise are key tools for preventing obesity at any age. Kids can benefit from lifestyle changes (not—I repeat, not—low-calorie diets that deprive them of energy and set them up for failure) that can turn them into fat-burning instead of fat-storing machines. The principles I outline throughout this book work for the entire family, and the battle against excess fat must be waged as a family. With the right tools and parental encouragement and support, we can create a generation of kids who will learn from their parents and be winners in the Fat Wars.

6

IT'S ALL ABOUT BALANCE

By now, it should be clear that becoming over-fat and reversing that process are highly specialized actions. Becoming fat and getting lean are complex hormonal actions our bodies have developed over millennia to ensure our survival. But when it comes right down to it, the process all begins in our head, and ends up in front of the refrigerator, as we make our choices about what to eat each day, when we'll eat it, and how much we'll put on our plates (for some of us, this is all we think about).

Our food is made up of both micronutrients (vitamins, minerals, and enzymes) and macronutrients. The latter—carbohydrates, dietary fats, and dietary proteins—contain the energy (in the form of calories) that our bodies run on, and the fats and proteins provide the structural materials our bodies need to rebuild, replenish, and replace our cells on a day-to-day basis. For a food to be high in a particular macronutrient (protein, carbohydrate, or fat), that macronutrient must dominate the food's caloric value.

For instance, many people mistakenly recommend the consumption of nuts and beans as sources of protein. This is very misleading, since nuts are actually quite low in protein but extremely high in fat (although much of this fat is good for you). Beans (with the exception of soy) are also low in protein and are high in carbohydrates.

Nuts, seeds, beans, and legumes	Fat%	Protein%	Carb%
Almonds (nut)	78	11	11
Cashews (nut)	73	11	16
Pumpkin (seed)	76	18	4
Sesame (seed)	76	12	12
Coconut (seed)	86	4	10
Garbanzo (bean)	11	22	67
Kidney (bean)	1	26	73
Lima (bean)	1	24	75
Split pea	1	26	73
Soy (legume)	47	38	15

Another example can be seen with a so-called high-protein food like steak. Commercially available (grocery-store purchased) sirloin steak contains only 29% protein, with the major macronutrient being fat at 71%. In fact, commercial beef should be labeled as a high-fat and moderate-protein food. Unfortunately, most of the fat in commercial grain-fed beef is also the harmful kind—saturated—unlike natural-grass-fed beef. (See Grass-Fed and Free Range: The Best Way to Eat Meat, pg. 71.) Natural grass fed beef contains certain fats that are actually allies in the Fat Wars. In nature, things quickly change. The protein content of noncommercial, undomesticated sources of meat such as venison (wild deer) or elk contains almost 82% protein (the major macronutrient), with a minimal fat content of 18%.

Now, calories are certainly part of the Fat Wars equation. Protein and carbohydrates contain 4 calories per gram; a gram of fat has 9 calories. If we consume more calories through food than we expend in energy, then we'll store those extra calories as fat. An active adult needs to eat between 1,600 and 2,500 calories a day to avoid loss of lean body mass. Obviously, some foods are more energy-dense than others: an apple, which is mostly water and fiber plus carbohydrates, has fewer calories than sirloin steak, which contains a lot of dietary proteins and dietary fats.

But in the Fat Wars, what you eat (and when you eat it) is just as important—if not more—as how much you eat. Throughout this book, I repeatedly stress the importance of eating like cavemen. We have inherited a living machine from our hunter-gatherer ancestors, a body designed to run best on a diet of wild game and unprocessed fruits, vegetables, nuts, and seeds. If we give it a fuel made up solely or primarily of carbohydrates and fat, for example (as in a typical North American diet), that machine won't run optimally, even if it has the requisite number of calories. Similarly, if we cut out certain nutrient groups—going on a fat-free diet, for example—we cheat it of a vital part of its ideal fuel and spare parts, and hormonal havoc ensues. Without the right types of fuel, in the right proportions, we run the risk of developing modern-day diseases and conditions such as: heart disease, diabetes, high cholesterol, high blood pressure or hypertension, stroke, infertility, certain cancers, immune dysfunction—and obesity.

Below, I profile the macronutrients that contain the energy we need to carry out the daily tasks of optimal living. I also discuss water and fiber. Although these two substances contain no calories, they are vital, if often overlooked, allies in the Fat Wars, and your diet should contain generous amounts of both. In the next section, I'll show you exactly how to combine these micronutrients into a high-octane fuel system that will ensure your body runs like a lean, mean, fat-burning machine.

Dietary Protein: Nature's Building Blocks

Your body is the site of a constant battle waged between two opposing forces: anabolic and catabolic. The first is the process of bodily renewal. The second is the process of bodily breakdown. The day your catabolic forces override your anabolic forces is the day you begin to die, at least on a cellular level. In other words, if you break down faster than your body can repair itself, you're in for a rough ride!

This elegant dance between catabolism and anabolism is one of the key factors to sustaining life. And protein plays a leading role (pun intended) in that dance. Every minute of every day, your body rebuilds, replaces, and replenishes about 200 million cells—that's almost 300 billion new cells every day. The raw materials your body uses to regenerate itself are called amino acids, and they are found only in protein.

Carbohydrates can supply the energy needed to build these body proteins, but they don't supply the actual raw building materials. Only protein (and certain fats) can do that. In other words, the adage "you are what you eat" is especially true when it comes to protein. (And, perhaps not surprisingly, protein is second only to water as the most plentiful substance in the body. Well over half your body's dry weight is protein.) Twenty-two amino acids are considered biologically important. Eight of them are considered essential, because the body cannot produce them and must obtain them from food. The liver can then synthesize the other fourteen amino acids from these original eight.

Protein synthesis, or the creation of new proteins from simple amino acids, is one of our most vital anabolic processes. When we are young, protein synthesis runs very efficiently, so we are predominantly anabolic. As we age, however, our catabolic metabolism begins to exceed our anabolic metabolism, and the body's ability to construct protein starts to slow. This is one of the reasons we lose muscle tissue and gain body fat with advancing age. And it's one of the reasons protein plays such a pivotal role in the Fat Wars.

On May 23, 2002, researchers from Ohio State University reported the discovery of a new amino acid—number 22. Prior to this, scientists had believed that there were only twenty-one natural amino acids—the key building blocks. This scientific finding suggests that there are probably more of these biological building blocks to be found.

Protein sets up the proper hormonal chain reaction necessary for fat loss and builds fat-burning muscle. Consumed with every meal, it increases your level of alertness and helps elevate your resting metabolic rate, even while you sleep. Protein also increases thermogenesis, or the body's ability to burn calories as heat: a high-protein meal will generate up to 40% more heat (and, therefore, burn many more calories) than will a high-carbohydrate meal. Research also shows that protein meals increase oxygen consumption at a rate two to three times higher than high-carbohydrate meals, indicating a much greater increase in the metabolic rate. Protein is also the main stimulator of the fat-burning hormone glucagon, which works in opposition to insulin, allowing the body to use fat as a fuel source instead of storing it as extra padding. The equation goes something like this:

- Dietary protein = stimulation of glucagon

- Glucagon secretion = stimulation of hormone-sensitive lipase (HSL), the fat-mobilizing enzyme

- HSL = fat loss.

A diet rich in protein contributes to greater gains in muscle during resistance training than does a high-carbohydrate diet—and more muscle equals more fat-burning capability. In fact, adding muscle (I'll show you how in Section III) can actually reverse the negative fat-storing effects of insulin resistance.

Higher-protein meals (with adequate good fats) are also more satisfying, filling you up more effectively than a high-carbohydrate meal, and consequently decreasing hunger.

If we are what we eat, we also are what our ancestors ate—and our ancestors ate a lot of protein. We are genetically predisposed to a diet composed of roughly 30% lean protein. In order to win the Fat Wars, then, we need to eat like our ancestors.

Not All Protein Is Created Equal!

Some of the best sources of lean dietary protein include chicken breasts, egg whites and whole eggs (preferably from free-run chickens), turkey breast, cold-water fish, seafood, isolated cross-flow microfiltered whey, and lean meats like wild game and tenderloin cuts (preferably from grass-fed animals). Good non-meat sources include organic yogurt, organic cheese, organic cottage cheese, fermented soy (in the form of tofu, miso, or tempeh), and, of course, high-quality soy-protein isolates.

With the exception of soy products, it can be difficult to get adequate protein from plant-based sources like nuts, beans, peas, or corn. A sizable portion of dietary proteins from vegetables is never absorbed by the body because fiber in these foods binds to the protein, making it biologically unavailable.

As you will learn in the next section, I highly recommend consuming five nutrient-dense but calorie-sparse meals a day, each of which should contain at least 30% protein, and two of which should be consumed as liquid protein shakes made with high-quality, high alphalactalbumin, cross-flow, membrane-extracted whey-protein isolates (see Appendix I for recommended brands). Whey isolates are the highest-quality, most bioavailable proteins ever discovered, and are therefore the best form of protein to support increased anabolism. Whey also offers many other benefits, such as increased antioxidant protection, hunger control, increased metabolism, cancer prevention, heart-disease prevention, and more. See Section II for some delicious shake recipes.

WHAT ABOUT RAW EGGS?

We've all witnessed the scene in *Rocky* when Balboa guzzles those raw eggs down before his run. Yuck! But since eggs are such high-quality proteins, wouldn't drinking them raw make sense? When you cook eggs (especially scrambled or fried) the heat causes oxidative damage to the cholesterol in the yolk. It is only oxidized cholesterol that can cause problems in our blood vessels. Egg yolks contain some of nature's most synergistic nutrients, which offer almost unprecedented health benefits (don't forget that the yolk of the egg is what contains the vital life force). The problem occurs when we consume the egg white raw. Raw egg whites contain a protein called avidin, which is a very powerful enemy of the B vitamin biotin. When uncooked, avidin is able to bind to biotin tightly, making it unavailable to the body. Cooked eggs, on the other hand, change the structure of avidin, making it susceptible to digestion and unable to interfere with the intestinal absorption of biotin.

So instead of consuming your eggs raw, try cooking your eggs by soft-boiling them or lightly poaching them. This way you minimize the damage to the cholesterol in the egg.

Dietary Fats: Your Surprise Fat Wars Allies

What if I told you that every morning I eat a tablespoon of pure oil? Surprised? I do.

You're probably thinking, "Oil's pure fat, right? And 1 tablespoon of oil has at least 120 calories! Is he nuts? What kind of Fat Warrior is this guy?"

Don't put down the book. Not all dietary fats (or fatty acids) make you fat! (If they did, then maybe low-fat diets would be more successful.) In fact, some of them—the fats, that is—will actually help you lose fat. And in order to win the Fat Wars, paradoxical as it may seem, you're going to have to get over your fat phobia. Let me tell you why fat—the right kind of fat—is a strategic ally in the Fat Wars.

In moderation, body fat is essential to life and health. As I discussed in Chapter 1, you always need some on hand for your body to burn as heat (thermogenesis). Our cell membranes, the covering that surrounds each cell, are made primarily of fat. The brain is nearly 60% fat. Maintaining proper heart rhythm requires the right balance of fat. Building bone density and strength also depends upon the right kinds of fat. And, get this: you need fat to burn fat. In fact, fat (the good stuff) should make up about 30% of your diet in the Fat Wars.

Good Fat? Bad Fat? Isn't Fat All the Same?

Not by a long shot. And knowing the difference between the different types (and structuring your diet accordingly) can make or break you in the Fat Wars.

You may have heard the terms "monounsaturated," "polyunsaturated," and "saturated" thrown around when people talk about fat. But what do they mean? Basically, they're variations on a structure: fats are composed of chains of carbon atoms with hydrogen molecules filling the available bonds. The type of fat depends on the length of those chains, the nature of bonds between the carbon atoms, and the number and arrangement of the hydrogen atoms attached to the carbon chain. But don't worry about the technical stuff—I'll break it down below.

The good

Unsaturated fats, as their name may suggest, aren't full: they have openings where more hydrogen atoms can fit in. The more space available for hydrogen, the more biologically active the fat is, and the more places it can go—besides your fat cells.

Monounsaturated fats (MUFA) have room for two hydrogen atoms, since they contain one (mono) double bond with two carbon atoms double-bonded to each other.

Polyunsaturated fats (see "And the Essential," below), on the other hand, have room for four or more hydrogen atoms because they contain two or more double-bond pairs. Both monounsaturated and polyunsaturated fats are important for overall health.

Consuming high amounts of MUFAs helps ward off cardiovascular disease and diabetes. These fats also act as antioxidants, mopping up the free radicals produced as the body oxidizes the sometimes bad LDL cholesterol. You can find MUFAs in olive, canola, and high-oleic safflower oil. They are also abundant in almonds and avocados. Add MUFAs to your arsenal of fat-fighting weapons—but remember, they are still fats, and thus are high in calories (9 per gram, like all fats). As you add MUFAs to your diet, eliminate calories from harmful fats and high-glycemic carbohydrates.

The bad

Saturated fats are full of hydrogen atoms and have a molecularly straight structure that allows them pretty much direct access to your fat cells (kind of like an arrow hitting a bull's-eye). The body can manufacture its own saturated fats, and doesn't need us to ingest them to get what it needs. They're pretty much useful to the body only as fuel—and we all know how much extra fuel we already carry in the form of stored fat. In excess, saturated fats can contribute to obesity, cardiovascular disease, certain cancers, and insulin resistance. Saturated fats indirectly cause insulin resistance by virtue of their damaging effects on muscle tissue. They accomplish this by causing minute microscopic breaks in the outermost layer of the muscle cells where the insulin receptors are located. If insulin cannot dock onto its receptors on muscle cells, then it will have to redirect any excess glucose toward our fat cells (if our glycogen reserves are full). These damaged insulin receptors also cause an unhealthy backup of insulin in the blood, which almost always becomes extra body fat.

By limiting your consumption of saturated fats, you can improve muscle-cell activity, increase your fat-burning rate, and reduce the deposit of fatty acids in your cells.

What foods contain saturated fats? They are found in high concentrations in grain-fed beef and dairy products, so choose lower-fat or leaner versions of these when you do consume saturated fat. They're also found in coconut oil, palm oil, and kernel oil (although coconut and palm oil do offer many health benefits as well).

The ugly

Trans fats are artificially altered fats. They've been chemically transformed through heat and hydrogenation (adding extra hydrogen molecules) to give the foods that contain them a longer shelf life. Those foods are some of the worst enemies in the Fat Wars: fried foods, margarine, and bakery products (bread, crackers, chips, cookies, pies, doughnuts).

Unfortunately, altering once-healthy, biologically active fats means that the end product (known in some circles as "Frankenstein fat") is even more easily incorporated into your eagerly waiting fat cells. And because our bodies don't recognize trans fat easily, such fat can cause hormonal havoc, including closing down our fat-burning machinery. Trans fats have also been shown to increase insulin, decrease testosterone, reduce energy metabolism, increase bad cholesterol, and inhibit immune function. Stay away at all costs.

And the essential

Remember that tablespoon of oil I down every morning? It contains a mixture of oils—flax, evening primrose, borage, pumpkin, fish, and currant-seed—high in omega-3 (alpha-linolenic acid or ALA) and omega-6 (linoleic acid or LA) fatty acids, also known as essential fatty acids (EFAs).

The "essential" officially means that the body cannot synthesize these fatty acids on its own and must get them from the diet. But these valuable fatty acids are also absolutely essential for health. Make them part of your fat-fighting arsenal.

These two fats (ALA and LA), along with—believe it or not—cholesterol, supply the building blocks of various structures within the body, including cell membranes and the raw ingredients that form the structures of the eyes, ears, brain, sex, and adrenal glands. They help detoxify the body, burrowing deep within to carry oil-soluble toxins to the skin's surface for elimination. They regulate traffic in and out of cells, ensuring that viruses, germs, and other hostile substances stay out, while cell proteins, organelles, enzymes, and genetic material stay in. They also help keep insulin functioning properly, help form red blood cells, and help make joint lubricants.

Omega-3 fatty acids, moreover, are essential for normal growth and may play an important role in the prevention and treatment of coronary artery disease, hypertension, arthritis, cancer, and other inflammatory and autoimmune disorders. Omega-3 fatty acids are particularly plentiful (in their activated form called EPA and DHA) in cold-water fish such as salmon, mackerel, herring, and trout, as well as algae.

And EFAs—yes, fats—ensure that we burn fat. They help increase the rate at which we burn fat by increasing the overall amount of oxygen utilized by the cells to produce energy as well as turning on the necessary switches on our genes that enhance overall fat burning. They also increase insulin efficiency and metabolic rate. As well, they are the precursors to a powerful group of hormone-like messengers called eicosanoids, a subgroup of which, called prostaglandins, can help slow insulin secretion and increase glucose tolerance.

By making both monounsaturated and polyunsaturated fats our main sources of dietary fat, we can substantially reduce unwanted fat stores.

BATTLING BODY FAT WITH CLA

Still not convinced that eating fat can help you lose fat?

Conjugated linoleic acid (CLA), a natural polyunsaturated fat found primarily in beef and milk (more in organic grass-fed varieties), has been shown in many studies to have powerful fat-loss potential.

In a recent study, presented in the *International Journal of Obesity* in August 2001, abdominally obese men who received CLA showed significant decrease in abdominal diameter after four weeks of supplementation (compared to a control group). None of the participants altered eating or exercise habits during the study.

In another study, presented in the December 2000 *Journal of Nutrition*, forty-seven people who supplemented their diets with CLA lost an average of 6 pounds of fat each over a twelve-week period.

The study indicated that approximately 3.4 grams of CLA per day is a good enough level for obtaining beneficial body fat reduction. Dr. Michael Pariza, a researcher who conducted CLA studies with the University of Wisconsin-Madison, found that when a group of seventy-one overweight dieters stopped dieting, and gained back weight, those who supplemented with CLA were more likely to gain muscle instead of fat. This is great news since statistics show that rebound weight gain after dieting is mostly in the form of body fat.

Below I have summed up some of the research on CLA over the last couple of years. CLA has been shown to:

- *Decrease excess abdominal fat (**visceral adiposity**):* Abdominal fat is the most unhealthy fat on the body. It predisposes us to heart disease, diabetes, and many other health complications. Fortunately tummy fat also happens to be the easiest body fat to lose (since it is a little more metabolically active than other fat). CLA imparts much of its body fat reduction in this area.

- *Aid in muscle growth:* As you are well aware of by now, muscle tissue dictates the overall metabolic rate—increasing your fat burning potential.

- *Increase metabolism:* This is very positive for those suffering from hypothyroidism (low thyroid) and other lowering metabolic disorders.

- *Increase insulin sensitivity:* A major condition in body fat accumulation is insulin resistance. By enhancing insulin sensitivity you may be able to not only prevent adult-onset diabetes, but control the rate at which fat accumulates in fat cells.

- *Reduces food-induced allergic reactions:* Since food allergies can be at play when weight loss becomes difficult, this can be of help to thyroid patients.

- *Boost immunity:* Many obese individuals have compromised immune systems. Cancer is an endproduct of compromised immunity. Many studies show CLA's potential benefits in the area of cancer prevention.

> • **Lowers blood fats:** Many obese and over-fat individuals have elevated cholesterol and triglyceride levels. CLA has been shown to help reduce these substances, which would allow for greater heart health.
>
> *See the Reference section for recommended sources.*

Eat fat like your ancestors

If you took an up-close look at one of the average North American's fat cells, you'd see that it stored about 50% MUFAs (the good), 30 to 40% saturated fatty acids (the bad), and only 10 to 20% polyunsaturates—or the essentials.

That's a far cry from what we would find if we were able to compare our fat cells to those of our hunter-gather ancestors. They evolved on a diet much lower in saturated fat than ours, and one that contained roughly equal amounts of omega-6 and omega-3 fats.

In the past century and a half especially, our consumption of fats has changed radically. The modern vegetable-oil industry sources its products from seeds rich in omega-6 fats. Modern agriculture emphasizes grain feeds rich in omega-6 fats. These food-processing and animal-husbandry practices have dramatically decreased the omega-3 fat content in many foods: green leafy vegetables, animal meats, eggs, and fish. The result is an upset in the balance between omega-6 and omega-3 fatty acids. Whereas the optimum ratio between the two should be one to one for the brain and four to one for the body's lean tissues, we're at a level of about twenty to one. That's too high, and can lead to health problems (overconsumption of omega-6 is linked to an increase in certain cancers and an increase in obesity). For this reason I suggest supplementing your diet with steam-distilled (no PCBs or mercury toxicity) cold-water fish oil (high in activated omega-3s). Fish-oil supplementation is also important because many people have trouble converting the omega-3 fatty acid ALA into EPA and DHA (its active forms). See the Appendix for recommendations.

GRASS-FED AND FREE-RANGE:
THE BEST WAY TO EAT MEAT AND EGGS

If ever there was proof that carbohydrates make you fat, just take a look at how feedlots fatten up cows for slaughter: they feed them as much grain as possible, instead of the grass that forms cattle's natural diet.

Similarly, the mass-produced eggs we find at the supermarket are the product of a chicken feed that bears little resemblance to chickens' more natural diet of vegetables high in omega-3 fats, insects, grass, fresh and dried fruit, and small amounts of corn. But animals fed a modern-day diet don't just get fat: they also yield meat and eggs severely imbalanced when it comes to omega-6 and omega-3 fatty acids.

The grain-fed beef we eat and the eggs we buy at the supermarket have omega-6 to omega-3 ratios that no longer resemble those in nature. Whereas free-range, natural-fed chickens produce eggs that have a ratio of one and a half to one, the average mass-produced egg has a ratio of twenty to one. After two hundred days in the feedlot, grain-fed cattle have omega-6 to omega-3 ratios exceeding twenty to one—much, much higher than the recommended ratio of three to one of grass-fed beef.

One of the easiest ways to balance EFA levels, then, is to switch to organic, free-range eggs and organic, grass-fed beef—these contain EFA ratios that our caveman-like genetic structures can recognize. As an added bonus, these products contain no hormones, antibiotics, or other chemicals. Finally, grass-fed beef is leaner than its grain-fed counterpart. See the Appendix for recommended sources.

Carbohydrates: Simply Complex

Here's a riddle: What's the difference between a baked potato and a quarter-cup of white sugar?

When it comes to your body's insulin response, the answer is surprising: there is no difference.

No, I'm not denying that eating a baked potato is better for you than eating sugar right out of the bowl! What I am saying, though, is that both foods are carbohydrates, and your body breaks down all carbohydrates into simple sugars like glucose. It doesn't particularly care where they come from. Sugar is sugar is sugar. And sugar, as I have discussed throughout the *Fat Wars Action Planner*, triggers an insulin response: the more sugar, the more insulin. Since the body can't use its stored fat as fuel when there's too much insulin in the bloodstream, eating too many carbohydrates spells victory for the dark side in the Fat Wars.

Carbohydrates come almost exclusively from plant sources, including grains, vegetables, and fruits. In highly processed forms, carbohydrates become white flour, white sugar, corn flour, and syrups, which are used to make the breads, pastas, cookies, and sweets we love so much. Carbs can be classified according to the rate at which they break down in the body: the ones that give up their sugars quickest are "high glycemic," while those that take longer to break down are referred to as "low glycemic." Not surprisingly, low-glycemic carbs eaten in moderation are our allies in the Fat Wars. (More on the glycemic index below).

Carbohydrates provide approximately 90% of the world's food supply. The top ten plant-based carb sources are wheat, maize, rice, barley, soybeans, cane sugar, sorghum, potatoes, oats, and cassava. Without these plants, the Earth could not feed its present 6 billion residents or the anticipated population of 12 to 15 billion people forecast for the next century. If agriculture gave us anything, then, it was an easily grown, calorically dense mass diet that could be stored, shipped, and processed in hundreds of different ways.

Although agriculture provides us with a handy way to feed the Earth's population, it may also have given us a diet incompatible with our genetic makeup. Remember, humans today share 99.9% of their genetic code with our hunter-gather ancestors, a code that was developed well before the advent of agriculture.

Between ten and twenty thousand years ago, there was a mass extinction of large mammals throughout Europe, North America, and Asia. To survive, our hunter-gatherer ancestors needed to expand their diets. Slowly, they abandoned a diet of predominantly wild meat, fruits, vegetables, and nuts (the same foods our present genes have adapted with) to take up entirely new dietary and activity patterns. For the first time, grindstones and crude mortars appeared in the archaeological record in the Near East. This was the beginning of humanity's use of cereal grains for food.

According to Dr. Loren Cordain, a professor of exercise physiology at Colorado State University in Fort Collins, Colorado, and a well-respected expert in the area of Paleolithic nutrition, this was a turning point in human evolution. We had evolved as hunter-gatherers, and our adaptive qualities weren't compatible with this new carbohydrate-based diet. The consequences became apparent: reduced body size (from which we have only recently recovered) and the appearance of cardio-vascular disease, cancers, diabetes, high blood pressure, and bone diseases, all characteristic—like obesity—of a sedentary population and carbohydrate-based diet.

As I discussed in Chapter 2, we are carbohydrate junkies: carbohydrates, many of them of the highly processed and/or high-glycemic variety, make up 50% of the average North American's diet. As a result, we pump out a lot of insulin, spelling the end to fat-loss goals and wreaking havoc on the body. The equation goes something like this:

- Dietary high-glycemic carbohydrates = stimulation of excess insulin

- Excess insulin secretion = stimulation of lipoprotein lipase (LPL), the fat storage enzyme

- LPL = fat accumulation

You already know that high insulin levels help make you fat. But they also damage the cardiovascular system by promoting the division of arterial smooth muscle cells, leading to clogged arteries and arterosclerosis. Over time, high insulin levels can lead to insulin resistance and eventually Type II diabetes.

The Fat Wars Glycemic Index

To keep blood-sugar (and therefore insulin) levels low and thereby begin our victory in the Fat Wars, we need to return to a diet typical of our hunter-gatherer ancestors. High-glycemic carbs were almost unheard of forty thousand years ago, unless our ancestors were lucky enough to come across a beehive. In such cases, the many stings would have been well worth the pleasure received from the sweet treat of honey.

There's definitely a place for carbohydrates in our diet; in fact, up to 40% of it should be made up of *low-glycemic* carbs. The foods at the bottom of the food chain, the unprocessed fruits (especially from the berry family) and vegetables that are high in fiber and water, are among the lowest on the glycemic index.

Obviously, in terms of the Fat Wars (and your health), the best carbohydrate choices are in the low-glycemic group. Restock the refrigerator and pantry to emphasize them—and ditch the refined breads, breakfast cereals, baked and mashed potatoes, white rice and rice cakes (yes, so-called diet food is in fact fat's friend), toaster waffles, Tater Tots, and French fries. Eat only small quantities of high-glycemic foods, and combine them with dietary proteins and fats in a meal. (But remember, even too much of the low-glycemic foods can make you fat!) In Section II (Fueling Your Body on Fat Wars) you will find a detailed Fat Wars Glycemic Index. Make it one of your greatest weapons in the Fat Wars. Please visit www.fatwars.com for updates.

A Natural Way to Slow Starch Digestion?

Specific inhibitors of animal alpha amylase (the enzyme that helps turn starch to sugar), were discovered in plants, particularly wheat and beans, as early as the 1940s. Interest in such inhibitors developed because controlled reduction of starch digestion theoretically could improve carbohydrate tolerance in pre-insulin diabetics and aid in weight control.

In 1974, J. John Marshall and Carmen M. Lauda purified a proteinaceous inhibitor of alpha amylase from kidney beans (*phaseolus vulgaris*), which they named Phaseolamin. In vitro (laboratory) research on Phaseolamin concluded it was a specific alpha amylase inhibitor.

The study also found that "a partially purified inhibitor, with increased specific activity, is stable in human gastrointestinal secretions, slows dietary starch digestion in vitro, rapidly inactivates amylase in the human intestinal lumen, and, at acceptable oral doses, may decrease intraluminal digestion of starch in humans." Based on this positive research, a number of companies began to reexamine use of amylase inhibitors for reducing starch digestion in diabetics and for weight control.

Pharmachem Laboratories, a major U.S. supplier of nutritional supplement ingredients, recently introduced Phase 2 (Phaseolamin 2250), the first standardized, non-stimulant starch neutralizer, extracted from a portion of the white kidney bean.

To demonstrate the effectiveness and safety of a standardized bean extract, Pharmachem recently sponsored some of the first human pilot trials at the University of Scranton. In a double-blind, placebo-controlled, crossover pilot study of eleven adult human subjects, starch absorption averaged 66% less in the group taking Phase 2.

> A European weight-loss study of sixty human subjects showed that those on Phase 2 lost an average of 6.45 pounds in thirty days, compared to those on placebo, who lost less than 1 pound, on average. Those participants on Phase 2 also lost, on average, more than 10% of body-fat mass, more than 3% in waist circumference, and measurable percentages off their hips and thighs. There was no loss of lean body mass, and personal evaluation of the participants showed good tolerability, with no adverse side effects. Of course a product like this should only be used for specific cheat days and not as a means to consume every carbohydrate in sight. For Phase 2 product recommendations, see Appendix.

Liquid Candy—and Other Dangerous Goods

If you really want to drive lots of calories into your fat cells, down a soft drink loaded with sugar, caffeine, and phosphorous.

The average soft drink contains 7-8 teaspoons of sugar—that's 7-8 times more sugar than your body is programmed to handle at any one time. The National Soft Drink Association in the United States (yes, there is such an organization) reports that the average American guzzled back the equivalent of seven hundred 12-ounce cans of pop (that's 7,000 teaspoons of sugar) in 2001. Given these numbers, it's easy to see why so many of us are in hormonal havoc. The pop we drink elevates insulin to sky-high levels, making us fat.

It also makes us addicts. The caffeine in pop is highly addictive, ensuring that we keep refilling our super-size cups. A 950-milligram serving of one of the leading colas contains between 98 and 125 milligrams of caffeine, enough to get us really hooked. Kids may be at even greater risk because, although they weigh less, they can down a big drink as if it were water. And since we experience caffeine withdrawal symptoms (like fatigue, headaches, malaise, anxiety, and depression) for a few days when cutting back on pop, very few of us withdraw: we just keep on filling up our liquid-candy containers.

"That's okay," you may be thinking, "I only drink diet sodas."

Think again. Most artificial sweeteners can affect your health just as negatively as sugar (and in some cases even more so). Sugar substitutes didn't exist when our bodies were evolving over the last hundred thousand years. Our bodies don't know what to do with them other than treat them as a type of sugar. Laboratory tests confirm that artificial sweeteners can boost insulin by fooling the body into thinking the sweetener is sugar. And remember, insulin causes our bodies to switch into fat-storage mode. When insulin is stimulated, it looks for sugar. When it can't find any real sugar from these substitutes, it ends up going after our blood sugar, causing us to experience an energy decline and a fat-storage increase.

If that weren't enough, the USFDA and other health organizations have been bombarded with numerous reports linking aspartame use to seizures, dizziness, visual impairment, disorientation, ear buzzing, tunnel vision, muscle aches, numbness of extremities, pancreas inflammation, headaches, high blood pressure, eye hemorrhages, and more.

So, if you want to win the Fat Wars, ditch the soda—regular *and* diet—in favor of clear filtered water. Give yourself a few days to get over the withdrawal symptoms, and you'll be home free.

Drink the Right Stuff

Although water has no caloric value, I include it in this discussion of micronutrients because, next to oxygen, it's possibly the most important thing you can put in your body to sustain life. It will also form a key part of your Fat Wars strategy.

We are made up mostly of water: one-quarter of bone tissue, three-quarters of the brain and muscle tissue, and more than 80% of the blood and lungs are made up of this vital substance. Without it, we'd shrivel up and die.

Without water, we'd have no energy. That's because water is imperative in the breakdown of adenosine triphosphate (ATP), our body's universal energy source. As I discussed in Chapter 1, to get energy, our bodies must first convert the carbohydrates, dietary fats, and dietary proteins we eat into ATP, which can then be used as energy. That process occurs in the mitochondria, tiny biochemical factories in our cells (mitochondria are also where the majority of our fat is burned as energy).

ATP is like an electrical source: nothing in our body runs without it. But if ATP is the electrical outlet, then water is like a plug that connects that energy source to the body. That's because ATP must be broken down by water (in a process called hydrolysis, which means "water broken") in order to release its energy. In a nutshell, a low-water environment means inadequate energy production. Intensive exercise, for example, can cause a person to lose 5 to 8 pounds of body fluid through perspiration, evaporation, and exhalation. Studies show that for every pound of fluid lost, the efficiency with which the body produces energy drops significantly.

But that's not all. Water helps the body eliminate toxins, the waste products that accumulate in our systems. When your 30 billion fat cells release their fat as energy, they also evict tremendous amounts of fat-soluble toxins that lodged in that fat. Your system needs water to help detoxify these toxins before they can take up residence once more in your fat cells.

Water is also an antiaging substance. Aging is, in a way, a process of drying up. As we age, we experience a decline in cognitive function that F. Batmanghelidj, M.D., a leading expert in water biochemistry and the best-selling author of *Your Body's Many Cries for Water*, believes may be due to the loss of water from certain areas of the brain and body. Many so-called signs of aging, says Dr. Batmanghelidj, are also signs and symptoms of chronic dehydration: heartburn, dyspepsia, rheumatoid joint pain, back pain and migraine headaches, hypertension, old-age diabetes, colitis, dry skin, constipation, autoimmune diseases, and cholesterol buildup, to name a few.

Water may also be an important way to control hunger pangs. Many researchers believe that we have lost our biological ability to discern thirst from hunger, a condition exacerbated by age: somewhere in our evolutionary past, the signals for the two may have crossed wires. In other words, when you feel hungry, you may actually be thirsty. By keeping yourself properly hydrated, then, you can avoid false cravings for food.

"But I *do* keep properly hydrated," you may be thinking: "I drink lots of liquids—juice, coffee, tea, and sodas!"

Let me be very clear here: nothing can take the place of water, especially not beverages like coffee, tea, or soda which contain caffeine and can dehydrate you. Juices and soda, furthermore, usually contain lots of sugar, a key enemy in the Fat Wars. (For more on soda, see "Liquid Candy—and Other Dangerous Goods," above.) And don't even think about alcohol. The more of these beverages you drink, in fact, the more water you will need to help clear them from your system. And most of us don't drink enough water in the first place. You need a *minimum* of eight to ten glasses of pure, filtered water every day, more if you exercise. Are you getting enough?

Try to consume clean filtered water throughout the day. Drink the water in a closed container through a straw to avoid taking in excess air and feeling bloated. Make a commitment to drink nothing but water for one full week. If you find water too bland, add approximately one half lemon or lime (preferably organic) to every liter of water for taste. After a week you won't want to drink anything else.

Fiber and the Fat Wars

Fiber is found in the indigestible portion of plant foods: the skin, peel, stalk, seeds, hull, or germ. Its main roles are to absorb moisture in the body, add bulk to the feces, and act as fuel for the beneficial bacteria that live in your gastrointestinal system. Even though fiber is derived from carbohydrate sources, the body lacks the necessary digestive enzymes to break it apart and extract its calories, thus making it a true calorie-free food. Fiber from foods is shuttled through our intestines, where it acts either as a sponge or a mop.

There are two classes of fiber—soluble and insoluble—each of which offers its own unique health benefits. Virtually all vegetables, fruits, and grains contain mixtures of the two types, although one type always dominates.

Soluble fiber—the sponge—is found in oats, barley, peas, legumes, certain fruits, and psyllium (pronounced sil-e-um). This type of fiber forms a gelatinous mixture with liquid in the digestive system. In doing so, it can absorb some of the body's excess cholesterol. What gives soluble fiber its grand appeal in the Fat Wars, however, is its ability to slow the release of glucose into the bloodstream following a meal, thereby lowering our overall insulin response (and fat-storage mechanisms). Soluble fiber has also been shown in many studies to reduce risk of heart disease.

Insoluble fiber—the mop—is found in leafy vegetables, root vegetables, and whole grains. This type of fiber passes through our digestive tract largely intact. Insoluble fiber is responsible for supplying the bulk, or roughage, that keeps foods moving through the digestive system unobstructed (and keeping us regular).

Fiber also helps us feel full without added fat and calories. Studies have shown that 5 to 30 grams of fiber (either kind) per day can effectively reduce hunger, making fiber even more valuable an ally in the Fat Wars.

If, like most North Americans, you don't eat the recommended 30 to 50 grams of fiber a day, then the foods you eat most likely begin to putrefy within your body. (Nice, huh?) Without fiber, foods don't pass quickly enough through the intestines and colon. Instead, they create a backlog of chemical waste that can eventually poison you (a process referred to as autointoxication). Adequate amounts of fiber, on the other hand, keep the digestive system healthy and can greatly enhance your fat-loss goals.

The Insulin/Fiber Connection

Fiber exerts a powerful double whammy against body fat.

First, because fiber, as I noted, helps slow the release of glucose into the bloodstream following a meal, it can moderate the effects of various foods on insulin levels. Adding fibrous vegetables to a meal of higher-glycemic carbohydrates, for example, retards the speed at which the sugars from these foods enter the bloodstream (this is not a reason for you to eat cake with a touch of lettuce with every meal). In other words, fiber, in a sense, turns higher-glycemic foods into lower-glycemic versions of themselves, thus lowering their insulin response and ultimately hampering the body's ability to store fat.

Second, insulin needs to bind to special receptors on muscle and fat cells to exert its metabolic actions. Certain soluble fibers, like beta-glucan (discussed below), have been shown to upgrade insulin-receptor sensitivity. When the insulin receptors in muscle are high, they are correspondingly low in the fat cells, and more sugars are diverted to muscle cells instead of turning into fat in the fat cells.

SOURCES OF FIBER	
Food	**Amount of fiber (in grams) in a 100 gram (3.5 ounce) serving**
Bread	
bagel	2.1
bran bread	8.5
pita bread (white)	1.6
pita bread (whole wheat)	7.4
white bread	1.9
Cereals	
bran cereal	35.3
bran flakes	18.8
cornflakes	2.0
oatmeal	10.6
wheat flakes	9.0
Grains	
barley, pearled (minus its outer covering)	15.6
cornmeal, whole grain	11.0
cornmeal, de-germed	5.2
oat bran, raw	6.6

Food	Amount of fiber (in grams) in a 100 gram (3.5 ounce) serving
rice, (brown)	3.5
rice, (white)	1.0-2.8
rice, (wild)	5.2
wheat bran	15.0
Fruits	
apple (with skin)	2.8
apricots (dried)	7.8
figs (dried)	9.3
kiwifruit	3.4
pears (raw)	2.6
prunes (dry)	7.2
prunes (stewed)	6.6
raisins	5.3
Vegetables	
beans	
baked (vegetarian)	7.7
chickpeas (canned)	5.4
lima, cooked	7.2
broccoli, raw	7.7
Brussels sprouts, cooked	2.6
cabbage (white) raw	2.4
cauliflower, raw	2.4
corn, sweet, cooked	3.7
peas with edible pods, raw	2.6
potatoes, white, baked, w/skin	5.5

Food	Amount of fiber (in grams) in a 100 gram (3.5 ounce) serving
sweet potatoes, cooked	3.0
tomatoes, raw	1.3
Other	
corn chips, toasted	4.4
nuts	
almonds, oil-roasted	11.2
coconut, raw	9.0
hazelnuts, oil-roasted	6.4
peanuts, dry-roasted	8.0
pistachios	10.8
tahini	9.3
tofu	1.2

Source: Provisional table on the dietary fiber content of selected foods (Washington, D.C.: U.S. Department of Agriculture, 1988).

BETA-GLUCAN: A POWERFUL WEAPON IN THE FAT WARS

Oats contain one of nature's richest sources of a special soluble fiber called beta-glucan. Several studies have shown that the greater the intake of beta-glucans, the greater the reductions in blood cholesterol (especially LDL, or bad cholesterol).

Researchers believe that beta-glucans lower cholesterol by transforming themselves into a viscous gel in the stomach. This gel is able to bind to bile acids—which contain excess cholesterol—and increase their rate of excretion. More than fifty clinical studies show the cholesterol-lowering ability of oats, while many other studies point to beta-glucan's ability to help with diabetes, hypertension, and, where the Fat Wars are concerned, obesity.

Beta-glucans help with fat loss by lowering the insulin response after a meal in both non-insulin-dependent diabetics and healthy subjects. More than a dozen published studies show that oats, consumed as oat bran, oatmeal, or isolated beta-glucans, can reduce both fasting and post-meal blood-sugar and insulin levels. A 1997 study published in the journal *Diabetes Care* showed that meals containing 8 to 10% beta-glucan were able to reduce glycemic responses by as much as 50% after a meal.

Studies also show that meals containing a sufficient supply of beta-glucan can greatly raise levels of the "feel-full" hormone CCK. Perhaps that's why oatmeal ranks as one of the top foods when it comes to feelings of fullness. It may also come as no surprise that oats contain the highest protein content of all the common grains. Including approximately 3 grams (the amount found in 1-1/2 cups of cooked oatmeal, 3/4 cup of uncooked oatmeal, or three packets of Quaker Instant Oatmeal) of beta-glucan in your daily diet may thus prove beneficial in your own Fat Wars. If you choose, you can also consume beta-glucans in a pure supplemental form—cutting out any additional calories or carbohydrates found in the oat bran or oatmeal (see the Appendix for recommended beta-glucan supplements).

YOUR BODY CHEMISTRY CHEAT SHEET

This is an additional section for referral purposes only. Throughout the *Fat Wars Action Planner*, I have discussed the various hormones that regulate your body's ability to burn or store fat. Your hormonal system has the power to send either positive messages (conducive to fat burning) or negative messages (conducive to fat storage) to your body's cells. And that system, to a very large extent, is under your direct control: it works according to the nutrients you feed it, the amount and quality of your exercise, and your stress levels. Treat your hormones well, and they will prove your most valuable asset in the Fat Wars.

Here's a handy summary of your body's key hormones (most of which I have discussed in the previous chapters, plus some extras) and how they affect your battle with body fat.

INSULIN

What is it and how does it work?	Friend or foe?	Strategy for fat burning
• Secreted by the beta cells of the pancreas. • Stimulated by carbohydrate (and, to a lesser extent, protein) intake. • Regulates sugar metabolism, promotes glucose utilization and protein synthesis (the manufacture of new tissues), and the formation and storage of fats. • Deposits glucose and amino acids into muscles and is therefore essential to muscle development, growth, and energy. • Converts glucose to glycogen within the muscles and liver. • Stimulates the storage of body fat from dietary fats and carbohydrates via the stimulation of the fat-storing enzyme lipoprotein lipase (LPL).	• Friend (most of the time) when there are low-glycemic foods in the system. • Converts any excess glucose to body fat via LPL. • High insulin levels inhibit the breakdown of stored body fat for fuel. • High levels can cause hypoglycemia (extremely low blood sugar), inducing extreme tiredness and insatiable hunger. • Insulin resistance and hyperinsulinemia (excessively high insulin levels) can lead to Type II diabetes. Both can cause decreased insulin function, leading to excess fat storage and possible heart problems. • Excess insulin can convert into pre-fat substances called triglycerides.	• Moderate your consumption of carbohydrates, especially highly processed ones that enter the bloodstream quickly. • Eat balanced meals every 2.5 to 3.5 hours to maintain balanced glucose levels. • Moderate coffee and alcohol intake: they have insulin-stimulating properties. • Exercise regularly. Exercise allows your body to absorb almost thirty times more glucose than it can at rest—independent of insulin. • Consume protein and essential fats at every meal, since these foods help control insulin's response to glucose. • Stress less. Excess stress can lead to excessively high insulin by stimulating stress hormones that elevate blood-sugar levels.

GLUCAGON

What is it and how does it work?	Friend or foe?	Strategy for fat burning
• Opposing hormone to insulin, secreted by the alpha cells of the pancreas. • Stimulated by protein intake. • Breaks down liver glycogen to maintain blood-sugar levels in the brain. • Initiates the breakdown of body fat by stimulating the fat-releasing enzyme hormone-sensitive lipase (HSL). • Stimulated through increased exercise after a certain level of glycogen has been depleted.	• Friend. It keeps blood-sugar levels from falling too low. • Converts excess amino acids from protein (not used by the body) into glucose (via gluconeo-genesis). • Inhibited by high insulin levels. If you can keep the two in balance, glucagon will stimulate fat release from your cells.	• Don't skip meals, exercise too much, or restrict calories too severely. • Make sure your body has a steady supply of high-quality protein throughout the day. • Remember that high blood-sugar levels will stop glucagon—and therefore fat burning—cold.

HUMAN GROWTH HORMONE

What is it and how does it work?	Friend or foe?	Strategy for fat burning
• Released by the anterior pituitary gland in the center of your brain in steady rhythms throughout the day and night.	• Friend. It helps the body recover after resistance training and increases lean body mass (muscle).	• Approximately 80% of HGH is released during the first few hours of sleep. Go to bed early and get a sound sleep, ensuring a deep-sleep

HUMAN GROWTH HORMONE *continued*

What is it and how does it work?	Friend or foe?	Strategy for fat burning
• Regulates growth and repair and stimulates body-fat breakdown.	• Helps decrease stored body fat by freeing it up as an energy source by inhibiting LPL activity.	phase from 11 p.m. to 2 a.m.
• Stimulates the release of specialized hormones called insulin-like growth factors (the most famous of which is IGF-1).	• Is considered to be one of the body's most potent antiaging hormones.	• Engage in regular, strenuous resistance exercise.
• Considered to be one of the most potent fat-burning hormones.	• Is the most potent anti-obesity agent ever discovered: it restores metabolic rate to that of our youth.	• Avoid high-glycemic foods, especially before exercise and bedtime.
• Can be greatly stimulated through intense exercise (especially weight training).	• An excess of HGH can cause abnormalities in bone growth and increase the incidence of Type II diabetes.	• Take a natural HGH precursor-called a secretagogue-before training, after training, or before bedtime.
• Inhibits LPL.		• Sleep in complete darkness to optimize melatonin production.
• Is blunted by high blood-sugar and insulin levels, high cortisol levels, and a hormone called somatostatin.		

MELATONIN

What is it and how does it work?	Friend or foe?	Strategy for fat burning
• Produced (as light diminishes) by the pineal gland in the center of your brain. • Stabilizes and promotes normal sleep and daily bodily rhythms. • Is one of the most powerful antioxidants produced in the body. • Has been shown to increase the life span of various animals by about 20%.	• Friend. Important in the repair and regulation of the body's immune systems. • Needed to help stimulate prolactin, which increases immune response during sleep. • Needed for the body to produce sufficient HGH. • Many people who take melatonin supplements have commented on an increase in the vividness or frequency of dream activity.	• Go to bed at a reasonable hour: melatonin production occurs during the early-morning hours of deepest sleep. • Sleep in as dark an environment as possible to avoid any light interference. • Consume high-tryptophan foods (see Chapter 3). • Commercially available in supplements of 2.5 or 3 milligram tablets, but many researchers believe that smaller dosages (0.5 to 1 milligram) are just as effective at regulating sleep.

PROLACTIN

What is it and how does it work?	Friend or foe?	Strategy for fat burning
• A protein hormone produced in the anterior pituitary, closely related to growth hormone.	• Friend. Helps modulate several aspects of immune function.	• Get adequate sleep: prolactin is secreted after approximately 3.5 hours of continuous

PROLACTIN *continued*		
What is it and how does it work?	**Friend or foe?**	**Strategy for fat burning**
• Also synthesized and secreted by immune cells, the brain, and the pregnant uterus. • Stimulates mammary-gland development and milk production in mammals.	• High dopamine levels can greatly suppress prolactin levels. • Agents and drugs that interfere with dopamine secretion or receptor binding lead to enhanced prolactin secretion.	melatonin secretion. • Some individuals may need almost 6 hours of continuous prolactin production to ensure optimal immunity, which suggests we may need almost 9.5 hours of total sleep.

CORTISOL		
What is it and how does it work?	**Friend or foe?**	**Strategy for fat burning**
• A steroid hormone released from the adrenal cortex (the outer membrane) in response to stress. • Referred to as a gluco-corticoid—a hormone involved in carbohydrate metabolism. • Released by the adrenal gland in times of stress (illness, traffic jam, teen tantrum, *dieting* ...)	• Foe. It destroys precious, fat-burning muscle in its quest for quick fuel by breaking down amino acids to form glucose. • In excess amounts, destroys muscle tissue. • Greatly increases blood-sugar levels and is always followed by a high-insulin response. • Can cause insulin resistance.	• Change your perception of reality. All stress is the same, whether real or imagined. • Don't diet. • Don't exercise too much. • Ensure you have a steady supply of high-quality protein in the diet.

CORTISOL *continued*		
What is it and how does it work?	**Friend or foe?**	**Strategy for fat burning**
	• Suppresses immunity by decreasing the production of specialized immune cells called lymphocytes (especially T cells) and antibodies.	• Eat every 2.5 to 3.5 hours to maintain balanced blood-sugar levels.

TESTOSTERONE		
What is it and how does it work?	**Friend or foe?**	**Strategy for fat burning**
• A steroidal hormone produced by the Leydig cells in male testes, and in lesser amounts by the adrenal gland near the kidneys (in both men and women), and the ovaries in women. • Precursor to estrogen in both men and women. • Needed to build and repair muscle tissue and burn body fat.	• Friend—if adequate levels are maintained. • Foe—if excess levels convert into dihydrotestosterone (DHT)—the powerful metabolite of testosterone. • Testosterone supplements are a great treatment for erectile dysfunction in men and low sexual desire in women.	• Ensure adequate levels of good fats in the diet (see Chapter 6). Low-fat diets contribute to low testosterone levels. • Exercise regularly with weights. • Eat adequate amounts of high-quality protein: higher-protein diets have been correlated with increased levels of testosterone. • Keep stress in check. High cortisol output degrades testosterone levels.

TESTOSTERONE *continued*

What is it and how does it work?	Friend or foe?	Strategy for fat burning
	• Adequate levels build strong muscles, bones, and ligaments; increase energy; and ease depression. • Low levels can cause fatigue, irritability, depression, aches and pain in the joints, thin and dry skin, osteo-porosis, weight loss, and the loss of muscle tissue leading to fat gain.	• Take stinging nettle to avoid excess testos-terone binding to SHBG. • Take stinging nettle and/or saw palmetto and Pygeum if you are con-cerned about high DHT levels. • Take the bioflavonoid chrysin if you are con-cerned about excess conversion (aromatiza-tion) of testosterone to estrogen (estradiol-E2). • If you are a woman, you may want to get off the pill! Recent evidence shows that the pill is responsible for lowered female testosterone levels. • If a physician recom-mends testosterone, ask for natural testosterone. • Women and men may see an increase in testos-terone by supplementing with DHEA.

ESTROGEN

What is it and how does it work?	Friend or foe?	Strategy for fat burning
• A steroid hormone produced in the ovaries and, to a lesser extent, the adrenal glands in women, and produced in men in the testes (in much smaller amounts than in women). • Affects over 300 different functions in the body—from building bones to strengthening the heart. • As women age, estrogen production from the ovaries and glands declines. • Can be produced in the fat cells. • Scientists now suggest that estrogen also works on regulating the brain. • Men's estrogen levels may actually increase instead of decrease with age, which is now thought to be one of the reasons that twice as many women are afflicted with Alzheimer's as men.	• Friend. Balanced levels in men's and women's bodies encourage a healthy libido, improve brain function, protect the heart, and strengthen the bones. • Foe: Excessive levels can lead to the suppression and reduced activity of testosterone—leading to a loss in muscle and a gain in body fat. • High levels in women can lead to estrogen dominance. • High levels in men can lead to an enlarged prostate, diabetes, and a higher incidence of heart disease and cancer.	• Obesity, pesticides, nutritional deficiencies, prescription medications, and excessive alcohol intake can all raise a man's estrogen levels. • Specific extracts of cruciferous vegetables called indoles-diindolylmethane (DIM) and indole-3-carbinol (I3C) enhances the liver's ability to metabolize estrogen into beneficial metabolites. This nutrient is especially good for women experiencing estrogen dominance. • Take stinging nettle to block the enzyme aromatase, which converts testosterone into estrogen. • If a physician recommends HRT, ask for natural estrogens. • Women (and some men) may want to look into natural progesterone (see below) if on HRT.

ESTROGEN *continued*

What is it and how does it work?	Friend or foe?	Strategy for fat burning
• Unlike the popular myth, estrogen is not a single hormone but instead a group of several different but related hormones. These include: • Estrone (approximately 10% to 20% of circulating estrogens) • Estradiol (approximately 10% to 20% of circulating estrogens) • Estriol (approximately 60% to 80% of circulating estrogens)		

PROGESTERONE

What is it and how does it work?	Friend or foe?	Strategy for fat burning
• A steroid hormone produced by the ovaries and the adrenal glands in women and, in smaller amounts, in the testes and the adrenal glands in men.	• Friend—if kept in balance. Low levels lead to the condition of estrogen dominance. • Progesterone depletion is now thought to cause many of the menopause symptoms suffered by women in a peri-menopause state.	• Topically applied natural progesterone cream has shown to aid dramatically in the relief and possible elimination of many menopause symptoms.

PROGESTERONE *continued*		
What is it and how does it work?	**Friend or foe?**	**Strategy for fat burning**
• One of its most important functions is in the female reproductive cycle. • It prepares the lining of the uterus for implantation of a fertilized egg, then helps to maintain it during pregnancy. • It can convert into estrogen or testosterone, as your body needs it. • Plays an important role in brain function (often called the "feel good hormone").	• If using a natural cream, be aware that since progesterone is highly fat-soluble, it stores itself in a woman's fat tissue, which over time can cause disruptions in the adrenal hormones, such as DHEA, cortisol, and testosterone. • Enhances mood and acts as an antidepressant. • Optimum levels can provide feelings of calm and well-being, while low levels can create feelings of anxiety, irritability, and even anger.	• Although the cream can offer tremendous benefits, it must be used very cautiously. • Beware of the synthetic version of progesterone called Provera, which can produce severe side effects, including increased risk of cancer, abnormal menstrual flow, fluid retention, nausea, and depression.

CHOLECYSTOKININ (CCK)

What is it and how does it work?	Friend or foe?	Strategy for fat burning
• A hormone that is secreted by cells in the duodenum (the first part of the small intestine). • It stimulates the release of enzymes from the pancreas and increases gall-bladder contraction and bowel motility. • Evidence shows that CCK acts on the brain as a satiety signal—"Thanks, I've had enough food for now."	• Friend. May provide help when it comes to preventing excessive food intake. • In animal studies, a rise in CCK is always followed by a large reduction in food intake.	• Can be stimulated by consumption of glycomacropeptides (GMPs)—low-molecular-weight protein peptides that exert an antibacterial and antimicrobial effect on our biochemistry. • In human studies, whey-protein glyco-macropeptides have been shown to increase CCK production by 415% within 20 minutes of ingestion. • Consume cross-flow microfiltered whey-pro-tein isolates with at least 20% GMPs once or twice a day.

LEPTIN

What is it and how does it work?	Friend or foe?	Strategy for fat burning
• A hormone produced by fat cells.	• Friend. The higher your leptin levels and the more active your leptin is, the higher your	• Eat regularly. Don't skip meals—this tactic leads to lower levels of leptin and changes in your

LEPTIN *continued*

What is it and how does it work?	Friend or foe?	Strategy for fat burning
• Appears to play an important role in how the body manages its supply of body fat. • It acts on nerve cells, mostly in the brain, to regulate body weight by increasing energy expenditure and decreasing food intake. • It signals the brain that no more fat storage is required, and (presumably) we stop eating. • Inhibits NPY synthesis and release (see below), stopping excessive cravings.	metabolism. • Obese people have a resistance to leptin, even though they sometimes produce greater levels of it than their thinner counterparts. • Can cause fat cells to self-destruct, thus eliminating their numbers.	thyroid hormones, and causes a slowdown in your metabolic rate. • Supplement with the mineral zinc. A 2001 study presented in the journal *Life Science* showed that obese individuals tend to have very low levels of zinc (referred to as hypozincemia), and that zinc treatment was able to increase leptin production by a whopping 142%.

OTHER PLAYERS

SEROTONIN

What is it and how does it work?	Friend or foe?	Strategy for fat burning
• A neurotransmitter (a chemical that transfers messages from one nerve or muscle cell to another).	• Friend—if kept balanced. • Foe—if levels are depleted, leading to carbohydrate craving and bingeing until levels are	• Consume adequate amounts of foods that contain tryptophan: chicken, milk, pineapple, turkey, soy, whey

SEROTONIN *continued*		
What is it and how does it work?	**Friend or foe?**	**Strategy for fat burning**
• Affects comprehension, memory, mood, body temperature, aggression, and appetite.	back up (and then some).	protein, or yogurt. • Stress less. Stress depletes serotonin faster than anything else. • Get adequate sleep. Serotonin levels are replenished during sleep. • Supplement with crave-free nutrients if needed (see Appendix I).

DOPAMINE		
What is it and how does it work?	**Friend or foe?**	**Strategy for fat burning**
• Also a neurotransmitter. • Affects brain processes that control movement, emotional response, and ability to experience pleasure and pain. • Its release causes feelings of reward and helps behavioral reinforcement. • Plays a role in cravings.	• Friend. Balanced levels decrease hunger and cravings and lead to enhanced metabolic rates. • Obese people have fewer receptors for dopamine, which causes them to eat more in an effort to stimulate the dopamine "pleasure" circuits in	• Consume plenty of high-quality proteins: dopamine's precursor comes from the amino acids phenylalanine and tyrosine. • Get sufficient sleep: neurotransmitters are replenished with deep sleep.

DOPAMINE *continued*

What is it and how does it work?	Friend or foe?	Strategy for fat burning
	their brains—just as addicts do by taking drugs. • Imbalanced dopamine activity can cause brain dysfunction and diseases such as central nervous system disorder, schizophrenia, and Parkinson's disease.	• Supplement with crave-free nutrients (see Appendix) and L-Tryosine (please get medical clearance first).

NOREPINEPHRINE (NORADRENALINE)

What is it and how does it work?	Friend or foe?	Strategy for fat burning
• Is a neurotransmitter of the sympathetic nervous system. • Also produced as a hormone in the adrenal glands. • Part of the fight-or-flight response • Is produced in response to short-term stress and is responsible for increased heart rate as well as blood pressure.	• Friend if not overstimulated, since it can increase the rate of body-fat breakdown. • Foe if overstimulated, as it can become catabolic, creating muscle breakdown, agitation, and insomnia.	• Perform regular bouts of high-ntensity resistance exercise. • Get plenty of high-quality sleep. • Supplement with thermogenic nutrients—especially those containing green tea extract with high levels of EGCG (see Appendix for recommendations).

NOREPINEPHRINE (NORADRENALINE) *continued*

What is it and how does it work?	Friend or foe?	Strategy for fat burning
• Other actions include increased glycogenolysis (the conversion of glycogen to glucose) in the liver, increased lipolysis (the conversion of fats to fatty acids) in fat cells, and relaxation of bronchial smooth muscle to open up the lungs and air passageways.		• Consume plenty of high-quality protein, as the amino acids phenylalanine and tyrosine are both precursors of norepinephrine. • You can also supplement (under the guidance of your physician) with the amino acids mentioned above.

BETA-ENDORPHINS

What is it and how does it work?	Friend or foe?	Strategy for fat burning
• Are neurohormones that are released from the pituitary gland in the brain. • Are a pleasure chemical responsible for relieving pain (analgesia) and producing euphoric feelings. • They're very addictive!	• Friend. Their release makes you feel euphoric and may even help build muscle and improve immunity. • The better shape you are in, the greater the beta-endorphin response and the longer the beta-endorphins stay elevated.	• Perform regular bouts of high-intensity resistance exercise. • Blood levels of beta-endorphins can increase in response to this form of exercise. • The better shape you're in, the greater the beta-endorphin response, and the longer they stay elevated.

BETA-ENDORPHINS *continued*

What is it and how does it work?	Friend or foe?	Strategy for fat burning
• They are many times more powerful than the drug morphine, and bind to the same receptors in the brain as morphine. • Are believed to be involved with muscle growth.	• They may help release extra HGH. • Many of the benefits of regular exercise (increased pain tolerance, greater appetite control, and reduced anxiety) are the result of beta-endorphin release.	

GALANIN (NEUROCHEMICAL)

What is it and how does it work?	Friend or foe?	Strategy for fat burning
• One of the most abundant neuropeptides in the brain. • It is thought to play a variety of roles, including regulation of the appetite and control of hormone secretion from the brain. • In times of famine, it stimulates fat storage (which is necessary under certain circumstances).	• Foe. It triggers fat cravings (and storage).	• Eat regularly. • Don't diet. • Don't eat highly saturated fatty foods, since these trigger galanin release, which further stimulates body-fat storage.

NEUROPEPTIDE NPY

What is it and how does it work?	Friend or foe?	Strategy for fat burning
• Is the most abundant neuropeptide in the brain. • Is known to be an extremely potent stimulator of feeding behavior.	• Foe. It causes insatiable cravings for carbohydrates, making it next-to-impossible to stay on a diet.	• Don't diet (especially by caloric restriction). • Since leptin inhibits NPY synthesis and release, it would be wise to consider supplementing with zinc.

section II

Fueling Your Body on Fat Wars

table of contents

Where you are and
where you need to be / 105

Working out your daily
caloric needs / 109

Eating principles summary
(timing and frequency) / 115

Nutrition factoids / 120

Ingredient factoids / 124

Fat war menus (recipes:
7- and 14-day cycles) / 130

DAY 1/MEAL 1
Organic Cooked Oats / 130

DAY 1/MEAL 2
Very Berry Shake / 131

DAY 1/MEAL 3
Roasted Turkey Sandwich / 131

DAY 1/MEAL 4
Banana Chocolate Shake / 132

DAY 1/MEAL 5
Baked Sole with
Coleslaw / 132

DAY 2/MEAL 1
Asparagus Omelet with Bagel / 133

DAY 2/MEAL 2
Banana Peach Shake / 133

DAY 2/MEAL 3
Spinach Salad / 134

DAY 2/MEAL 4
Protein Boost / 135

DAY 2/MEAL 5
Fat Wars Chili / 135

DAY 3/MEAL 1
Organic Muesli / 136

DAY 3/MEAL 2
Hawaiian Pineapple Delight / 136

DAY 3/MEAL 3
Fruit Salad with Cottage Cheese / 137

DAY 3/MEAL 4
Holiday Shake / 137

DAY 3/MEAL 5
Salmon Delight / 138

DAY 4/MEAL 1
Open=faced Egg Muffin / 138

DAY 4/MEAL 2
Carrot Top Shake / 139

DAY 4/MEAL 3
Roast Beef Sandwich / 139

DAY 4/MEAL 4
Protein Rush / 140

DAY 4/MEAL 5
Mandarin/Chicken Salad / 140

DAY 5/MEAL 1
Granola with Strawberries / 141

DAY 5/MEAL 2
Sweet and Sour Shake / 141

DAY 5/MEAL 3
Anytime Burrito / 142

DAY 5/MEAL 4
Blueberry Shake-it / 142

DAY 5/MEAL 5
Shrimp Stir-fry / 142

DAY 6/MEAL 1
Egg Breakfast / 143

DAY 6/MEAL 2
Orchard Blend / 144

DAY 6/MEAL 3
Mexican Marvel / 144

DAY 6/MEAL 4
Frozen Colada / 145

DAY 6/MEAL 5
A Real Steak Dinner / 145

DAY 7/MEAL 1
Berry Cottage Cheese / 146

DAY 7/MEAL 2
Protein Punch / 146

DAY 7/MEAL 3
Broccoli Soup and Chicken
Sandwich / 147

DAY 7/MEAL 4
Yogurt Delight / 147

DAY 7/MEAL 5
Tuna with Greek Salad / 148

DAY 8/MEAL 1
Muesli Delight / 148

DAY 8/MEAL 2
Really Good 4U
Cheese Whiz / 149

DAY 8/MEAL 3
Tuna Sandwich / 149

DAY 8/MEAL 4
Strawberry/Rhubarb Shake / 150

DAY 8/MEAL 5
Lamb with Wild Rice / 150

DAY 9/MEAL 1
Peanut Butter and Banana / 151

DAY 9/MEAL 2
Phyto Nutrient Delight / 151

DAY 9/MEAL 3
Super Chicken Soup / 152

DAY 9/MEAL 4
Kiwi/Banana Rama / 152

DAY 9/MEAL 5
Scallop Jambalaya / 152

DAY 10/MEAL 1
Spinach and Feta Eggs / 153

DAY 10/MEAL 2
Protein Dream / 154

DAY 10/MEAL 3
You Betcha—It's a Pizza! / 154

DAY 10/MEAL 4
Grapefruity / 155

DAY 10/MEAL 5
Steak Kabob / 155

DAY 11/MEAL 1
Poached Eggs "N" Cheese / 156

DAY 11/MEAL 2
Berry Orange / 156

DAY 11/MEAL 3
Egg Salad Sandwich / 157

DAY 11/MEAL 4
Chocolate Dreams / 157

DAY 11/MEAL 5
Salmon and Stuffed Pepper / 158

DAY 12/MEAL 1
7-Grain Hot Cereal / 159

DAY 12/MEAL 2
Frozen Blue / 159

DAY 12/MEAL 3
Shrimp Salad / 160

DAY 12/MEAL 4
Green Beret / 160

DAY 12/MEAL 5
I Yam a Steak / 161

DAY 13/MEAL 1
Yogurt Fruit Salad / 161

DAY 13/MEAL 2
Cran-Apple Fun / 162

DAY 13/MEAL 3
It's a Wrap / 162

DAY 13/MEAL 4
Veggie Protein Surprise / 163

DAY 13/MEAL 5
A Very Veggie Stir-fry / 163

DAY 14/MEAL 1
The Muse / 164

DAY 14/MEAL 2
Trail Mix / 164

DAY 14/MEAL 3
Shrimp and Miso / 165

DAY 14/MEAL 4
Tahiti Treat / 165

DAY 14/MEAL 5
Cajun Cod / 166

Fat Wars On The Town / 167

A Few More Points / 171

FUELING YOUR BODY ON FAT WARS

Where You Are and Where You Need to Be

Congratulations for making the commitment to finally win your Fat War. My first book, *Fat Wars: 45 Days to Transform Your Body*, opened many people's eyes to why they were having such a difficult time combating their wily fat cells. That book took thousands of North Americans (and still does) by the hand and led them on a forty-five-day journey to body transformation. The amazing reality was that the thousands of successful Fat Warriors realized by the end of their program that fat loss was not merely about body transformation, but really about a total life transformation instead. Once life-stripping fat is depleted from your body, you too will notice a life transformation by not only looking better and having more self confidence (although very important), but also feeling and performing better than you ever thought possible.

Fat Wars: 45 Days to Transform Your Body was only the beginning. It is a program designed to show you the importance of fat loss as oppose to just weight loss, but most importantly it is a program that shows you how to mobilize the fat you are now living with and finally incinerate it in your metabolically active tissues. *Fat Wars* showed you how to upregulate your metabolic rates and turn your biochemistry into one of a fat burner instead of a fat storer.

This section of the book will provide you with practical guidelines and tools that will set you up for continued success on the Fat Wars program. If you implement the Fat Wars eating principles (along with the Biocize™ exercise strategy in the next section), you will stimulate the proper hormonal environment conducive to fat burning, instead of fat storage. With the Fat Wars eating principles, each and every meal takes you one step closer to winning your Fat Wars. Remember, you are only as good as your last meal, hormonally speaking.

By following the outlined recommendations and meal plans, you will be be setting yourself up for one victory after another in the Fat Wars. You will not only learn how to implement a winning plan for losing unwanted body fat, but more importantly you will start to practice behaviors that will enable you to keep the fat off forever. The *Fat Wars Action Planner* provides you with easy-to-use guidelines and recipes that allow you to follow and enjoy the Fat Wars strategies, all the while tracking and measuring your success. The important thing to remember here is that Fat Wars is not another diet, but instead a new healthier way of living your life.

Let's Start by Evaluating Where You Are

Please honestly answer the following questions and record your score:

1. How many meals do you presently eat per day?

   1   2   3   4   5   6   7   8   9   10

2. What is the general timing between each meal? I eat approximately every ...

   1 hr. 2 hrs. 3 hrs. 4 hrs. 5 hrs. 6 hrs. 7hrs. 8 hrs. 9 hrs. 10 hrs.

3. When you finally eat your meals are they (size)?

3	2	1
Small	Medium	Large
(less than 300 cal.)	(more than 500 cal.)	(more than 1,000 cal.)

4. Identify the types of carbohydrates, proteins, and fats that you eat most of each day:

Carbohydrates:

3	2	1
mostly sugary and processed baked goods, highly processed goods	refined flours, white rice, white bread, and pasta	a variety of vegetables and fruits, legumes, and unprocessed grains such as oats, millet, kamut, quinoa, barley, etc.

Fats:

3	2	1
mostly margerine, vegetable oils, beef and chicken fat, cheese, pastries, doughnuts, chocolate bars, french fries, potato chips, etc.	processed sauces, convenience foods low-fat cheese, margarine, sauces and creamy salad dressings	organic butter, egg yolks, omega-3-rich foods such as: sardines, flaxseed, salmon, olive oil, canola oil, and a variety of nuts and seeds

Proteins:

3	2	1
bacon, hamburgers, pork ribs, chicken with crispy skin, hot dogs	whole milk, peanut butter, regular ground beef	lean meat, fish, organic milk, skinless chicken and turkey breast, low-fat cottage cheese, soy and whey protein, and legumes

5. You eat most of your carbohydrates:

3	2	1
in the evening	at mid-day	first thing in the morning

Score:

1. If your answer was 6 or higher, then your score = 10
   If your answer was 5 or lower, your score is = 1

2. If your answer was 4 hrs. or higher, then your score = 10
   If your answer was 3 hrs. or less, then your score is = 1

3. Record the score that corresponds with your answer.

4. Record the score that corresponds with your answer for carbohydrates, fats, and proteins.

5. Record the score that corresponds with your answer.

   Your final score:

   1. _____ +

   2. _____ +

   3. _____ +

   4. _____ +

   5. _____ +

   = _____ total score

Where You Need to Be

If your score was higher than 10 then you are in the position to benefit the most from the strategies outlined in this part of the book. The strategies will be focused around the Fat Wars eating principles, which helped tens of thousands of people transform their lives for the better. Please understand that it takes time, energy, and focus to change an old (unhealthy) habit. But once your body realizes what true healthy vibrancy feels like, I promise you will never want to go back to your old habits again.

Working Out Your Daily Caloric Needs

Since its inception, Fat Wars has helped many thousands of individuals just like you achieve their ultimate transformation goals. Within the last couple of years, I have received thousands of e-mails from people who followed the Fat Wars forty-five-day transformation plan with astounding success. The amazing thing is, that there were still a number of people who lost considerable amounts of their body fat, yet did not follow the caloric requirement method of the program. This is because when the majority of the Fat Wars recommendations are adhered to, even if the caloric requirement portion is not, will still allow you to convert your metabolism to one of a fat burner.

This is not to say, however, that you will achieve the same results as if you did follow the caloric recommendations outlined here. The main objective of Fat Wars is for you to change your life. And in order for you to achieve life change, you will have to become comfortable with your new Fat Wars lifestyle program so that you incorporate it into your daily life. In other words, the object of Fat Wars is to deliver a program that is not only workable in your life, but one that you can actually enjoy and look forward to. This means that if you are a person who *will not* under any circumstance follow a calculated plan of attack on your 30 billion fat cells by figuring out daily alloted calorie requirements, then you will have to find another method. And it has to be a method that you can work with (not to mention one that works with you) in order to see continual results. If you find yourself in this category, please try to follow as closely as possible the following method of meal design.

Fat Wars for Beginners

Follow the Fat Wars recommendations regarding exercise and eating smaller portions of food five times a day—all the while making sure each of your meals are metabolically balanced. The Fat Wars principle of consuming three solid meals and two protein shakes per day still applies here (you can also use some of the sample meal plans and recipes below to get an idea of how a Fat Wars meal is metabolically balanced). If you follow all of these suggestions, you can still lose a great deal of excess body fat, although from experience, those who use a daily plan of attack (by knowing ahead of time how much food they can consume) experience greater results. So if you are still not someone who has the patience to weigh your food and calculate your daily caloric allotment, that's okay. You can still make the Fat Wars Action Planner work for you by following these guidelines:

- Re-read Chapter 6 (or Chapters 6 through 8 in the original *Fat Wars: 45 Days to Transform Your Body*) or go onto the Fat Wars Web site at www.fatwars.com and click on the Fat Wars Fuel icon to find out what your best food choices are on the Fat Wars plan.

- Never let more than three and a half hours pass between meals.

- Eat five meals every day: three solid meals and two protein shakes. Each meal should contain protein (30%), essential fats (30%), and low-glycemic carbs (40%)—use approximate values pertaining to percentages. The last meal should be void of any high- or medium-glycemic carbs. Best results coming from various salads and stir-fries.

Attention night shift workers: You can use the principles outlined in this section to design your own Fat Wars Action Plan. As indicated above, the last meal you consume prior to sleeping should be void of any high- or medium-glycemic carbs.

Creating your Fat Wars meal the simple way:

- Meal timing is one of the most important elements when consuming a Fat Wars meal. If you follow the conventional method of eating two or three large meals a day, or even worse, skipping a meal or two, you will set into play fat storage with each meal due to unbalanced blood sugar levels with elevated insulin levels.

- Use a dinner-sized plate and visually divide it into three equal sections.

- Use the palm of your hand to determine the size for your protein element and make sure the protein portion is also about the thickness of your hand. This equates to approximately 3 ounces for a woman and 4 ounces of low-fat protein for a man.

- Place the protein in one of the sections on the plate. For example, you could eat a serving of chicken or turkey that's roughly the size of your palm.

- Fill the other two-thirds of the plate with a heaping portion of fresh fibrous vegetables or place vegetables on one-third of the plate and fruit on the other third. This becomes your carbohydrate portion. If your carbohydrate choice is a starch (and these should be used sparingly due to their higher glycemic rating) such as a sweet potato, rice, or beans, add only one-third more than the protein portion (1.3 to 1 ratio), and eliminate the fruit serving.

- For your fat source, sprinkle a small portion (approximately 1 tablespoon) of organic olive oil or flaxseed oil to the meal or simply add a few almonds.

The Fat Wars Meal Battle Strategy

Battling your fat cells with a proven strategy for success with the *Fat Wars Action Planner*, leaves nothing to chance. The following strategies success becomes magnified when you keep a daily journal of your battle plan. By charting one successful battle at a time (one meal at a time), you can better get a feel for what is working best for your body. This method becomes a strategic plan of attack on your 30 billion fat cells, and as it is based on thousands of testimonials, it is your best chance for success.

As you have probably figured out by now, protein is the four-star general that leads the army in the Fat Wars. By first figuring out your daily protein needs (in calories or grams), you will then be able to calculate the remaining calories or grams of the other two nutrients (fats and carbs). In order to receive a reliable assessment of your daily protein needs, you will first have to get a lean body analysis completed. If you do not have access to a body fat analyzer (I especially recommend the Futrex models because of their accuracy)—you can usually find one through your local gym or fitness center. Then use the body fat calculator on the Fat Wars Web site at www.fatwars.com to find your approximate body fat percentage. Although not as accurate as a professional method, the calculator is a close enough guideline to follow until you can secure a more accurate reading through bio-impedance or infrared technology.

Once you have determined your body fat percentage, take the number and multiply it by your present body weight (follow example below). Next, take the new number and subtract it from your present weight. The new number represents your lean (fat-free) body mass. Now you can calculate your daily protein requirements using the formula that best describes your activity level:

- **No Exercise**: $0.75 \times$ lean body weight (in pounds)

- **1 to 2 Workouts Per Week**: $1.00 \times$ lean body weight (in pounds)

- **Over 3 Workouts Per Week**: $1.15 \times$ lean body weight (in pounds)

- **If You Are an Athlete**: $1.25 \times$ lean body weight (in pounds)

The number that you get represents your daily protein requirement, in grams, on the Fat Wars plan. Take this number and divide it by five to arrive at the amount of protein allotted at each meal.

I'll use one of my clients, Lisa, as an example:

- Lisa presently weighs 150 pounds and carries 30% body fat. If I multiply 30% (which is equal to .30) by 150, I end up with the number 45, which represents the total amount of fat, in pounds she is carrying (.30 $\times$ 150 = 45 lbs.)

- Because fat is an inert substance, it doesn't require any protein, unlike our lean body mass. So next, I subtract the amount of body fat (45 pounds) from Lisa's present body weight (150 pounds) and I arrive at 105 pounds of lean weight.

- I then take 105 (Lisa's lean weight) and multiply it by 1.15 since Lisa has just started the Fat Wars Plan and is now working out 3 times a week. 105 $\times$ 1.15 = 121.

- The number 121 represents Lisa's total daily protein requirement in grams.

- Because she is following the Fat Wars plan and is now eating five times per day, Lisa now divides 121 grams by five meals to get 24 grams of protein per meal.

- Lisa would now make sure that each of her five meals throughout the day contains approximately 24 grams of protein.

After you have your total daily requirement of protein, you can easily figure out your total caloric allotment by looking at the **Daily Total Fat Wars Recommended Macronutrient Breakdown Chart** below. Simply look down the *protein* (*30%*) column until you find the number that represents your daily allotted protein requirement to the nearest one-hundredth (using the above example, Lisa would choose 120 g from the list as this is the closest amount to her daily needs). All the other figures in the corresponding line represent your daily needs. Everything is figured out for you. All you have to do is divide each amount by 5 to figure out your caloric and gram requirement for each meal (three solid meals and two protein shakes).

Daily Total Fat Wars Recommended Macronutrient Breakdown Chart

Based on 30% of calories from protein, 30% of calories from fat, and 40% of calories from carbohydrate

Caloric intake	Protein (30%)	Fat (30%)	Carbohydrate (40%)
1,200	90 g (360 cal.)	40 g (360 cal.)	120 g (480 cal.)
1,300	97.5 g (390 cal.)	43 g (360 cal.)	130 g (520 cal.)
1,400	105 g (420 cal.)	47 g (420 cal.)	140 g (560 cal.)
1,500	112 g (450 cal.)	50 g (450 cal.)	150 g (600 cal.)
1,600	120 g (480 cal.)	53 g (480 cal.)	160 g (640 cal.)
1,700	127.5 g (510 cal.)	57 g (510 cal.)	170 g (680 cal.)
1,800	135 g (540 cal.)	60 g (540 cal.)	180 g (720 cal.)
1,900	142.5 g (570 cal.)	63 g (570 cal.)	190 g (760 cal.)
2,000	150 g (600 cal.)	67 g (600 cal.)	200 g (800 cal.)
2,100	157.5 g (630 cal.)	70 g (630 cal.)	210 g (840 cal.)
2,200	165 g (660 cal.)	73 g (660 cal.)	220 g (880 cal.)
2,300	172.5 g (690 cal.)	77 g (690 cal.)	230 g (920 cal.)

Caloric intake	Protein (30%)	Fat (30%)	Carbohydrate (40%)
2,400	180 g (720 cal.)	80 g (720 cal.)	240 g (960 cal.)
2,500	187.5 g (750 cal.)	83 g (750 cal.)	250 g (1,000 cal.)
2,600	195 g (780 cal.)	87 g (780 cal.)	260 g (1,040 cal.)
2,700	202.5 g (810 cal.)	90 g (810 cal.)	270 g (1,080 cal.)
2,800	210 g (840 cal.)	93 g (840 cal.)	280 g (1,120 cal.)
2,900	217.5 g (870 cal.)	97 g (870 cal.)	290 g (1,160 cal.)
3,000	225 g (900 cal.)	100 g (900 cal.)	300 g (1,200 cal.)
3,100	232.5 g (930 cal.)	103 g (930 cal.)	310 g (1,240 cal.)
3,200	240 g (960 cal.)	106 g (960 cal.)	320 g (1,280 cal.)
3,300	247.5 g (990 cal.)	110 g (990 cal.)	330 g (1,320 cal.)
3,400	255 g (1,020 cal.)	113 g (1,020 cal.)	340 g (1,360 cal.)
3,500	262.5 g (1,050 cal.)	116 g (1,050 cal.)	350 g (1,400 cal.)

Remember to divide each number by 5 in order to get an accurate value of how many calories and grams of protein, fat, and carbohydrates to consume at each of your five meals. For the best results, you should try to hit these values as closely as possible each day.

Note: Please understand that Fat Wars is not a starvation diet plan in any way. The plan is based on lean body percentage and active tissue (lean body mass) caloric needs. There's no point taking in more calories than you are going to burn if your goal is fat loss. If you are a larger and more active participant than my example of Lisa, you will have a larger calorie allotment. The reverse is also true.

As your body transformation starts taking place, you will start to gain lean body weight and lose body fat. It is important to have your lean body mass checked every three months in order to gauge fat loss success and recalculate daily caloric and gram allotments. In essence, the more muscle you create on your frame, the more calories your body requires. Imagine that, a plan that actually increases your caloric amounts instead of lowering them over time.

> The reason the Fat Wars program is so effective is that it is hormonally designed and does not promote hunger, because the three macronutrients and blood sugar levels are balanced.

Eating Principles Summary (Timing and Frequency)

The key to optimizing energy levels, increasing muscle and burning fat is to fuel your body properly throughout the day. Equally important to your fat loss success is the timing and frequency of each of your *five* meals. Adhering to the "Fat Wars" eating principles as closely as possible will determine your degree of success on the program. I encourage you to follow the simple guidelines I provide and consult the Fat Wars glycemic index chart when making food choices.

The Fat Wars Eating Principles

The Fat Wars eating principles include:

- Eating *five* equal and calorically balanced nutrient-dense meals per day.

- Making sure that each of your *five* meals (including shakes) is as close as possible to the Fat Wars macronutrient profile of:

- *40% complex carbohydrates*: from low-glycemic carbohydrate choices including fruits and vegetables. These foods will ensure energy production, thyroid conversion, muscular repair, and will maintain a proper balance of insulin to glucagon for effective fat burning. Do your best to avoid heavy starches like processed flour contained in products such ad bread and commercial baked goodies. Also avoid cornmeal containing products (i.e., corn chips), pasta, and refined white rice.

- *30% lean proteins*: from lean high-bioavailable protein choices including: game meat (whenever possible), tenderloin, chicken breast, fish and seafood, organic plain yogurt, and cottage cheese. My protein choice for the Fat Wars shakes will come from the highest-quality whey (preferably high alphalactalbumin) isolates, soy isolates, or a mix of both whey and soy. These foods will help to increase your metabolic rate, regulate anabolic metabolism, and maintain a proper balance of glucagon to insulin (which will help to stimulate fat-burning enzymes).

- *30% healthy fats*: from healthy fat choices, including: foods that contain omega-3 fatty acids (cold-water wild fish, fish oil, flaxseed, flax oil, perilla oil, hemp oil, pumpkin seeds, and walnuts), omega-6 fatty acids (nuts and seeds, organic butter, egg yolks, and monounsaturated fats, such as olive oil and avocados) in moderation. Do your best to limit consumption of fatty cheese, beef fat, and lard, and *completely* avoid all food containing trans fatty acids, including margarine, French fries, potato chips, and commercial baked goodies.

• Make sure that *three* of your daily meals are in a solid form and two are in a liquid form (Fat Wars 40-30-30 protein shakes).

• Include plenty of good fats (omega-3 fatty acids, olive oil, almonds, and so on) in your diet each day.

• Consume an 8-ounce glass of water approximately twenty minutes before each of your five meals.

• Consume water as your beverage of choice, making sure to drink approximately *ten* glasses each day.

• Make sure to leave at least two hours between your last meal and bedtime. It is best not to eat after 8 p.m.

The Glycemic Index for Selected Foods

EAT MORE—10% TO 49%—LOW GLYCEMIC FOODS	
Grains:	
Barley	Whole-sprouted grains
Bran cereals	Whole-grain pasta, el denté
Muesli cereals (without dry fruit)	Kamut and quinoa pasta
Bulgur	Red basmati whole-kernel rice
Porridge oats	Spaghetti (whole-meal) el denté
Cooked oatmeal and bran	

Dairy:

Low-fat cottage cheese	Most (1%-whole) milk
Low-fat soy milk	Plain yogurt (no sugar added)

Nuts and Seeds:

Peanuts	Sesame seeds
Almonds	Sunflower seeds

Legumes:

Adzuki beans	Navy beans
Black beans	Soybeans
Black-eyed peas	Split peas
Butter beans	Haricot beans
Garbanzo beans	Kidney beans

Vegetables:

	Broccoli and Cauliflower
Artichokes	Peppers
Asparagus	Tomatoes
Celery	Dark leaf lettuces
Potatoes (sweet)	Yams

Fruits:

	Nectarines
Apples	Oranges
Apricots	Peaches
Berries	Pears
Cherries	Plums
Grapefruit	Strawberries

Beverages:

Green tea	Tomato juice
Unsweetened grapefruit juice	Unsweetened pear juice
Water	

EAT LESS—50% TO 69%—MODERATE GLYCEMIC FOODS

Grains:

Basmati rice	100% Whole-wheat bread
Brown rice	Pumpernickel bread
Buckwheat	Sourdough bread
Spaghetti (white)	Wild rice
Pita bread	Shredded wheat
Water biscuits	

Dairy:

Custard	Skim milk

Vegetables:

Beets	Yams
Carrots	Peas
Corn on the cob	Potatoes
Lima beans	

Fruits:

Bananas	Raisins
Grapes	Figs
Kiwifruit	Watermelons
Mangoes	Pineapples

Beverages:

Apple juice	Blackberry cherry juice
Blueberry juice	Orange juice

Sweeteners:

Unrefined raw honey	Organic unrefined brown sugar
Unprocessed black strap molasses	

EAT AT YOUR OWN RISK—70% TO 100%—HIGH GLYCEMIC FOODS

Grains:

Bagels	Pancakes
Breakfast cereals (refined, with sugar added)	Puffed rice
Corn chips	Shredded wheat
Cornflakes	Toaster waffles
Rice cakes	White bread
Crackers and crispbread	White rice
Doughnuts	Whole-wheat bread
French bread	Weetabix
Hamburger or hot dog bun	Muffin (commercially processed, white flour)
Pretzels	

Dairy:

	Chocolate syrups
Cool Whip	Chocolate Milk

Vegetables:

Cooked carrots	Parsnips
French fries	Sweet corn
Potato (baked)	

Fruits:

Banana (ripe)	Papaya

Beverages:

Carrot juice	Soft drinks and sports drinks

Sweeteners:	
Corn-syrup solids	Molasses
Honey	High-fructose corn syrup
Barley malt	Maltose

AVOID EATING—100% GLYCEMIC FOODS
Glucose, maltodrextin-based drinks

Nutrition Factoids

• **Filtered water**: It is imperative to teach your body to accept and enjoy water as the beverage of choice. Your body is 75% water, not 75% coffee, pop, juice, or any other beverage. According to biochemical water expert Dr. Batmanghelidj, M.D., somewhere through evolution our signals for thirst and hunger went awry. As we age, when our bodies become dehydrated, we misinterpret the thirst signals for hunger. I suggest drinking a full glass of filtered water twenty to thirty minutes before eating to replenish fluid and deal with confused thirst signals. Never wait until you are thirsty or have a dry mouth to drink water; by this time your body is already in a state of dehydration. Losing muscle mass as a result of dieting or aging will also contribute to intracellular dehydration, because a fat cell can hold only 15% water, whereas a muscle cell can easily hold 75%. Water is also essential to your elimination systems. As you deplete your fat-cell accounts, you also release the many toxins that were once held in your fat cells into your system. It is important to remove these toxins through effective elimination, and water is the essential nutrient to ensure this happens (along with fiber).

• **Organic whole food choices**: Even though it is not always stated, all ingredients are meant to be organic. This is for your own good. Organic foods supply an enhanced nutritive value to our bodies' structures and are as close as we are presently going to get to the way our ancestors ate. Organic foods are also free from unnecessary chemicals, preservatives, contaminants, and other harmful substances, for example pesticides, herbicides, and fungicides. A whole food refers to a natural, unprocessed food, for example, brown or long-grain rice, which contains the bulk of its fiber and essential micronutrients, instead of polished white rice, which does not. According to a study in the *Journal of Applied Nutrition*, the majority of organic fruits, vegetables, and grains have more than 90% more minerals than conventionally grown food.

• **Fruits and Vegetables**: It is important to consume a wide variety of fruits and vegetables for their phytonutrient- and alkaline-forming abilities. The wider the variety of rich colors you choose in these foods, the better. As fellow researcher and colleague Sam Graci, M.A., puts it in his best-selling book, *The Power of Superfoods*: "You have only to take advantage of these foods to unleash the enormous power they contain. Foods from your refrigerator, cupboard, or fresh-fruit bowl are the most powerful modulator of your body chemistry."

Please do your very best to purchase organic produce whenever possible.

Virtually any single fruit or vegetable listed below (or anywhere else in this book, for that matter) carries in it the potential of an abundance of chemical-like substances that offer health-promoting effects to your body. These phytonutrients are found throughout the entire fruit or vegetable, and especially in the skin and seeds. Some of these powerful chemicals are listed below:

• **Berries (especially blueberries), grape (seeds and skin), and red wine**: contain bioflavonoids, flavonoids, ellagic acid, anthocyanidins, and cis-resveratrol. These are powerful antioxidants that help protect our genetic structures (DNA), especially in the brain, and enhance the other network antioxidants. They also work to keep our blood vessels flexible and elastic, reduce inflammation, and help stop cancer formation.

• **Citrus fruits (including the pulp)**: contain monoterpenes that enhance liver enzymes, which detoxify carcinogenic substances.

- **Onions (yellow and red), yellow squash, shallots, red grapes, and sweet potatoes**: contain a bioflavonoid called quercetin that can inhibit tumor-stimulating enzymes, reducing cancer formation.

- **Broccoli, broccoli sprouts, Brussels sprouts, kale, cabbage, cauliflower, arugula, watercress**: contain sulforophane and indoles such as indole-3-carbinol and diindolylmethane (DIM), which neutralize carcinogens and alter the enzyme pathways that control estrogen production, favoring beneficial metabolites of estrogen that increase progesterone production and testosterone production and enhance fat burning. Indoles are also able to alter cancer formation by inhibiting PKC growth signals, which stop cancer cells from replicating.

- **Soybeans, soy sprouts, soy protein isolates (including transform+), miso, tempeh, tofu, bee pollen, green tea**: contain isoflavones (genistein, daidzein, and glycitein), glucosinolates, and protease inhibitors. These powerful nutrients are capable of deactivating excess sex hormone production (estrogen or testosterone) and lowering the risk of hormone-dependent cancers of the breast, cervix, uterus, and prostate.

- **Garlic, onions (including chives and shallots)**: contain allicin and allylic sulfides. These sulphur compounds are some of nature's most potent antioxidants and exert antibacterial, antifungal, and antiviral actions on the body. They have been shown to reduce the risk of stomach and colon cancer.

- **Tomatoes, spinach, lettuce, peppers, berries, and green-food concentrates (greens+ and transform+)**: contain carotenoids (alpha, beta, gamma, delta-carotene, lycopene, lutein, and zeaxanthin). These specialized color pigments can enhance immune system activity, balance blood-sugar levels, kill pathogens in our air, water, and food, and protect against stomach and colon cancer. Lutein and zeaxanthin prevent macular degeneration of the eyes.

- **Organic flaxseed and high-lignan flaxseed oil, whole grains, and sprouts**: contain lignans, which compete for estrogen receptors and therefore block excess estrogen, to reduce breast and prostate cancer.

- **Oatmeal and oat bran**: Oats contain a much-researched form of fiber called beta-glucan (see Chapter 6, Beta-glucan: A Powerful Weapon in the Fat Wars) that can help to decrease insulin response by increasing digestion time. Oats also contain the very important essential omega-6 fatty acid called gamma linolenic acid (GLA). GLA is able to form powerful hormone-like substances that enhance the body's fat-burning potential.

- **Apple fiber, whole grains, legumes, nuts, seeds, vegetables, fruit, and whole brown rice**: Help to eliminate excess toxins and waste from the body and enhance beneficial bacteria populations. They absorb excess bile and other cancer-causing substances; they prevent the reintroduction (reuptake) of estrogen into the body, thus improving estrogen balance, and they reduce excess cholesterol and balance blood-sugar levels.

- **High alphalactalbumin whey-protein isolate (proteins+)**: contains glutathione-enhancing precursors that help modulate immunity and aid in liver detoxification. Helps create an anabolic environment for enhanced muscle growth and fat loss. Contains serotonin and melatonin precursors that help balance moods, eliminate cravings, and induce optimum sleep. Nature's most bioavailable source of protein.

- **Game meat, grass-fed organic beef, and organic milk products**: contain the fatty-acid-conjugated linoleic acid (CLA) that helps deflate the body's fat cells, especially around the midsection. CLA has also been shown to be a powerful anticancer fat. Game meat and grass-fed beef, as noted in Chapter 6, contain much less saturated fat then commercial grain-fed beef, making them excellent bioavailable-protein and low-fat food sources.

- **Organic plain yogurt**: contains friendly GI bacteria called probiotics. These friendly bacteria aid in digestion, assimilation, and elimination of food. They reduce excess cholesterol, enhance overall immunity, and neutralize toxins, chemicals, and yeast throughout the intestines.

- **Flaxseed, flaxseed oil, hemp oil, organic borage oil, cold-water fish (sardines, salmon, mackerel) and cold-water fish oils**: contain omega-3 fatty acids, which are essential to our biochemistry, as the body must obtain them by dietary means. These good fats form hormone-like eicosanoids, which enhance cellular communication and aid in fat loss. They are also powerful anti-inflammatory and anticancer compounds.

Ingredient Factoids

• **Breads**: Any breads you choose on the Fat Wars plan should come from organic, whole, natural, sprouted grains and stone-ground whole-grain flours that contain pure water (no chlorine, fluoride, or tri-halomethanes), and only natural sweeteners. Sprouted grains offer superior nutrition and fiber to other forms of grain because, as a seed sprouts, the nutrients inside multiply many fold (please see box below). This also causes the food to change from an acid to an alkaline base.

SPROUTING VS. MILLING

General milling (or grinding) practices generate a substantial amount of heat that adversely affects the grain. This excess heat production oxidizes the kernel and causes loss of vital vitamins (B and E) within twenty-four hours. Most of the bran and germ is removed in milling to control rancidity. This allows most flours, including whole wheat, to have a longer shelf life.

If you want to consume grain, do so either in the form of stone-ground (as long as it is used within twenty-four hours of grinding) or sprouted.

You will notice that most of the breads listed here are from the Silver Hills line of breads. I have no affiliation with this company, but I do recommend them as a premier choice if you must eat grains, due to their high-quality organic ingredients and the fact that they use sprouted grains exclusively (you can visit them on line at: www.silver-hillsbakery.ca). When including bread in your daily diet, please try to limit consumption after meal three, due to bread's higher-than-normal glycemic ratings. Unfortunately, the majority of individuals overconsume highly processed white-flour products that have no nutritive value for the body. I have included healthy bread alternatives in various recipes here, to show that these food choices can be Fat Wars friendly.

• **Eggs**: You will notice that there are quite a few recipes using eggs in this action planner. Try to buy organic eggs or eggs from chickens reared on a high-omega-3 fatty-acid diet. When chickens consume feed that is fortified with essential omega-3 fats, their eggs contain higher-than-normal ranges of these beneficial fats. I have also listed shake recipes containing raw (organic) egg yolks. I do not recommend consuming whole raw eggs because the white of the egg contains a specific glycoprotein (protein-carbohydrate molecule) called avidin, which is not found in the yolk. Avidin binds to the B-vitamin biotin very specifically and tightly, and in doing so can cause biotin depletion, which can lead to serious neurologic disorders when it is consumed on a regular basis. Cooking deactivates avidin in the egg white.

Raw egg yolks (please read box below), on the other hand, offer many health benefits, including liver and brain support, because of their high natural lecithin levels. Lecithin is easily destroyed by low cooking temperatures. Lecithin is a powerful fat emulsifier that helps in the breakdown and transport of dietary fat. Many people are concerned with the amount of cholesterol found within the yolk. Research is proving that the total amount of cholesterol is not the important factor, but the amount of damaged or denatured cholesterol is.

When egg yolks are heated above 105°F, their vital life force becomes altered, causing structural changes in many of the yolks' elements, including cholesterol. The process of cooking causes the cholesterol component of the egg yolk to oxidize, in turn creating free-radical damage in the body. Our blood vessels only have receptors for oxidized cholesterol-which causes more plaque formation in our arteries.

For this reason, and because egg whites contain a good amount of iron (iron has the ability to further oxidize cholesterol), I do not recommend preparing eggs any other way than boiling, as in poached or soft, medium, and hard boiled. Scrambling or frying eggs creates a combined reaction with iron and heat to create excess oxidation of the cholesterol component of the yolk. Boiling eggs limits the destruction to the cholesterol component, and cooking egg whites alone eliminates the problem altogether.

• **Organic eggs**: contain lecithin and phosphatidyl choline, good fats that maintain brain function and enhance memory and mood. These fats also keep nerve membrane and brain cell membrane integrity intact. They also enhance liver function and help break down (emulsify) body fat. A sluggish liver can impede fat loss.

IMPORTANT: With eggs and all other raw foods from animals, there is a small possibility of salmonella food poisoning. The risk is increased for those who are pregnant, elderly, or very young and those with compromised or impaired immune systems. These individuals should avoid raw and undercooked animal foods.

There is very little risk for healthy individuals as long as you treat eggs and other raw animal foods carefully. Use only properly refrigerated, clean, unbroken, fresh, Grade AA or A eggs. Avoid mixing yolks and whites with the shell. Refrigerate broken-out eggs, prepared egg dishes, and other foods if you won't be consuming them within an hour.

• **Milk and milk products**: Even though I am not a big supporter of consuming an abundance of milk products, I do understand that many of you have grown up on these items and will not do without them. As in the examples you will find in the Fat Wars menu cycles, please use these products sparingly, and exclusively in organic form. The organic varieties offer a higher nutritional value to your body as well as elevated levels of the fatty-acid-conjugated linoleic acid (CLA), especially if the cattle have been reared on grass as opposed to grains.

THE CALCIUM CONNECTION

Ask almost anyone on the street where they get their daily fix of calcium, and most will reply, "Why, milk of course!" Yes, milk, does contain a fair amount of calcium. However, the amount of calcium contained in various foods is just part of the story when it comes to how your body uses calcium. Isn't it enough to know that when you eat cheese, you will also be consuming a great deal of calcium to keep your bones healthy and strong? No! The reason is that your body also uses calcium to balance excess acidity. As foods are digested, they leave behind either an alkaline or an acid ash or residue of sorts called the acid-base balance. If the majority of the foods consumed contain an acid ash—as do unsprouted grains, legumes, meat, fish, eggs, and let's not forget dairy products with hard cheeses leading the pack—then you will actually lose more calcium in your urine. However, if you have consumed enough alkaline-based foods—such as fruits and vegetables—to balance the excess acidity, then you'll retain calcium.

If you haven't got the picture yet, even if you consume copious amounts of high-calcium foods such as dairy products, you may end up losing bone mineral density (through calcium excretion) if you don't eat enough fruits and veggies. This is one of the reasons I advocate 40% of your diet coming from carbohydrates that contain alkaline, such as fruits and vegetables.

• **Game meats and grass-fed (free-range) meats**: Whenever possible, choose meats from animals that are reared in as natural an environment as possible, such as game animals and cattle left to graze on grass (please see Chapter 6, Grass-Fed and Free-Range: The Best Way to Eat Meat). Recommended grass-fed suppliers can be found in the Appendix.

• **Seeds and nuts**: Organic seeds and nuts offer us an unsurpassed way to obtain essential fatty acids the body uses to create energy, build cellular membranes, and create powerful hormone-like substances called eicosanoids, which among other things, help the body burn fat. (Please see Chapter 6, And the Essential on pg. 67.)

You will note that I have listed a lot of flaxseed and flaxseed oil as part of the protein shakes. Flaxseed and flaxseed oil contain nature's highest levels of omega-3 fatty acids. The problem today is that we consume way too many of the omega-6 variety of fatty acids. Modern estimates place our adult dietary ratio somewhere in the vicinity of twenty to one. Though experts disagree on the precise ideal ratio, most agree that it lies somewhere between one to one and four to one.

FOOD SOURCES OF EFA AND THEIR MESSENGERS

PG series	Fatty acid	Fatty acid family	Food sources
1	Linoleic	n-6	Sunflower, safflower, sesame, corn
1	gamma-linolenic	n-6	Primrose, borage, and black currant seed oil
2	arachidonic	n-6	Animal meat, milk, eggs, squid, warm-water fish
3	alpha-linolenic	n-3	Flax, canola, pumpkin, chia, walnut, Brazil nut
3	EPA	n-3	Cold-water fish, krill, algae (some)
3	DHA	n-3	Cold-water fish, krill, algae (some)

WHY BUTTER INSTEAD OF MARGARINE?

I am not exactly a fan of margarines. One of the main reasons is that a lot of margarines contain molecularly altered harmful fats called trans fats that are formed through the process of hydrogenation or other methods of adulteration. Margarines can be very high in trans fatty acids, though some members of the food industry have taken steps to reduce trans fatty acids in their foods. But margarines are not the only processed foods that contain these harmful forms of fat.

French fries, potato chips, chicken nuggets, deep-fried fish burgers, and doughnuts contain anywhere from 8 to 13 grams of trans fatty acids per serving. Doughnuts have been found to contain up to 13 grams of trans fatty acids. If a food lists "partially hydrogenated oil" on the label, it will also contain trans fatty acids. Some calculations have shown that an adult male consuming 145 to 250 grams of fat per day, which is not unheard of, might consume nearly 50 grams of this fat as trans fatty acids.

One of the problems with trans fatty acids is that they are solid at our bodies' own temperature, which causes our cells to become more rigid and inflexible. These fats have been shown in animal studies to easily cross the blood-brain barrier, which means they could end up as part of our nerve-cell membranes. What about butter? Butter, unlike most margarines, contains no trans fats. In fact, butter isn't that bad at all. Although butter is a saturated fat, its chemical structure is comprised of a short-chain (four-carbon) fatty acid called butyric acid. Butyric acid contributes to enhanced immunity and contains antimicrobial properties, which help protect us from viruses, yeasts, and harmful bacteria that reside in the gut. Due to its small molecular structure, butter does not require bile acids to be broken down in the stomach; it is absorbed directly into the bloodstream for energy production. This is one of the reasons that short-chain fatty acids like butter, consumed within reason, do not cause fat gain. So instead of avoiding butter, go ahead and use it sparingly—without guilt (but try to make it organic!).

FAT Wars Menus: Seven- and Fourteen-day cycles

The following Fat Wars menus will help you learn how to design a hormonally balanced Fat Wars meal. After figuring out your daily caloric requirements based on lean body mass and using the Daily Total Fat Wars Recommended Macronutrient Breakdown Chart, find the caloric amount that closest represents your needs and add or subtract a minor amount of the listed ingredient based on your needs. For instance, if you need 1,700 calories a day, then add more than the

1,600 calorie suggested amount but less than the 1,800 calorie category.

You will notice that two of the meals each day are based on protein shakes (either using a shaker cup or a blender). If you are unable to make blender-required shakes, please use alternate meal plan shake choices (i.e., using shaker-cup protein shakes and consuming nuts, seeds, fruit, vegetables, etc.) All shake recipes include protein. When mixing your shakes, always use water as the medium (for shaker cups, water levels are indicated on cup), unless otherwise specified. Although I have used a water measurement as a guideline, please adjust water to your desired consistency as everyone has their own preference. The measurement abbreiviations are as follows:

• S - one level scoop

• HS - one heaping scoop

Please note that all the recipes were developed and tested using proteins+™ but you may substitute with a high alpha whey isolate if you wish.

DAY 1/MEAL 1

Organic Cooked Oats

	1,600	1,800	2,000	2,200	2,400	2,600
Organic Oats, slow-cooking	½ cup	½ cup	⅔ cup	⅔ cup	¾ cup	¾ cup
Milk, 1%	¼ cup	¼ cup	⅓ cup	½ cup	⅔ cup	¾ cup
Strawberries, fresh	¼ cup	¼ cup	⅓ cup	½ cup	½ cup	⅔ cup
High alpha whey isolate (scoop)	1	1	1 ½	1 ½	2	2
Nuts, walnuts	½ oz.	⅔ oz.	¾ oz.	¾ oz.	¾ oz.	¾ oz.
Raisins, seedless	1 tbsp.	⅛ cup	⅛ cup	⅛ cup	⅛ cup	¼ cup

Directions: Place your portion of slow-cooking oats in a glass or ceramic bowl and add double the amount of boiling water to the oats. Cover with a lid and let sit for 15 minutes (or till desired consistency). Remove lid and add milk first and then all other ingredients. Mix all ingredients together and enjoy.

DAY 1/MEAL 2

Very Berry Shake

	1,600	1,800	2,000	2,200	2,400	2,600
Vanilla high alpha whey isolate (scoop)	1	1 ½ cup	1 ½	1 ½	2	2
Yogurt, plain low-fat	¼ cup	⅓ cup	⅓ cup	½ cup	½ cup	½ cup
Blueberries	½ cup	½ cup	⅓ cup	½ cup	½ cup	½ cup
Strawberries	⅛ cup	¼ cup	¼ cup	¼ cup	⅓ cup	⅓ cup
Blackberries	⅛ cup	¼ cup	¼ cup	¼ cup	⅓ cup	⅓ cup
Raspberries	⅛ cup	¼ cup	¼ cup	¼ cup	⅓ cup	⅓ cup
Flaxseed, crushed	1 tsp.	1 tsp.	1 ¼ tsp.	1 ¼ tsp.	1 ⅓ tsp.	1 ½ tsp.

Directions: In blender, place all ingredients except protein and flaxseed. Blend well until all berries are puréed. With blender on low speed, add protein and flaxseed and mix until blended (aproximately 10 seconds).

DAY 1/MEAL 3

Roasted Turkey Sandwich

	1,600	1,800	2,000	2,200	2,400	2,600
Turkey breast, light roasted	2 ½ oz.	2 ½ oz.	3 oz.	3 ½ oz.	4 oz.	4 oz.
100% whole-wheat stone-ground bread	2	2	2	2	2	2
Mayonnaise (organic)	½ tbsp.	¾ tbsp.	¾ tbsp.	¾ tbsp.	¾ tbsp.	1 tbsp.
Cranberry sauce, whole berry	1 ½ tsp.	⅛ cup	⅛ cup	⅛ cup	⅛ cup	¼ cup
Lettuce, green leaf	⅛ cup	⅛ cup	⅛ cup	⅛ cup	⅛ cup	⅛ cup
Tomato	1 slice	2 slices	3 slices	3 slices	3 slices	3 slices
Applesauce, unsweetened	⅛ cup	⅛ cup	¼ cup	½ cup	⅔ cup	¼ cup

Directions: Lightly toast bread. Mix mayonnaise and cranberry sauce together and spread over bread. Place turkey breast, lettuce, and tomato on one slice of bread and cover with the other. Applesauce may be eaten on its own or used for dipping sauce.

DAY 1/MEAL 4

Banana Chocolate Shake

	1,600	1,800	2,000	2,200	2,400	2,600
Chocolate high alpha whey isolate (scoop)	1 (S)	1 (S)	1 (S)	1 (S)	1 ½ (S)	1 ½ (S)
Banana, medium	½	½	½	¾	⅔	¾
Yogurt, plain low-fat	⅔cup	⅔ cup	1 cup	⅔ cup	1 cup	1 cup
Flaxseed, crushed	¾ tsp.	1 tsp.	1 tsp.	1 ¼ tsp.	1 ¼ tsp.	1 ½ tsp.

Directions: In blender, mix banana and yogurt together. Blend well. Add protein and flaxseed and blend for additional 10 seconds on low.

DAY 1/MEAL 5

Baked Sole with Coleslaw

	1,600	1,800	2,000	2,200	2,400	2,600
Sole	3 oz.	3 ½ oz.	4 oz.	4 ½ oz.	4 ½ oz.	5 oz.
Dill	1 tsp.	1 ¼ tsp.	1 ¼ tsp.	1 ¼ tsp.	1 ¼ tsp.	1 ⅓ tsp.
Olive oil	½ tbsp.	½ tbsp.	½ tbsp.	½ tbsp.	½ tbsp.	½ tbsp.
Lemon	⅛	¼	¼	½	½	½
Cabbage, green	⅛ cup	⅛ cup	¼ cup	⅓ cup	⅓ cup	½ cup
Cabbage, red	⅛ cup	⅛ cup	¼ cup	⅓ cup	⅓ cup	½ cup
Organic mayonnaise	¼ tbsp.	⅓ tbsp.	½ tbsp.	½ tbsp.	½ tbsp.	¾ tbsp.
Raisins	¼ cup	¼ cup	⅓ cup	⅓ cup	⅓ cup	⅔ cup
Pepper	½ tsp.	½ tsp.	⅔ tsp.	⅔ tsp.	⅔ tsp.	⅔ tsp.

Directions: Mix dill and olive oil together; brush over sole. Slice lemon and place over sole. Bake in oven at 325°F for 20 minutes, turning fish over halfway through cooking time. Chop cabbage. Mix mayonnaise with cabbage and add raisins and pepper.

DAY 2/MEAL 1

Asparagus Omelette with Bagel

	1,600	1,800	2,000	2,200	2,400	2,600
Egg, whole	1	1	1	1	2	2
Egg whites	3	4	5	4 ½	3	3
Asparagus spears	4	4 ½	6	6	6	6
Butter	⅓ tbsp.	½ tbsp.	½ tsp.	½ tsp.	¼ tsp.	½ tsp.
Milk, 1%	1 tbsp.	1 tbsp.	1 tbsp.	1 tbsp.	1 tbsp.	1 tbsp.
Bagel, organic multigrain	½	½	½	1	1	1
Pepper	½ tsp.	⅔ tsp.	1 tsp.	1 tsp.	1 tsp.	1 tsp.
Tomato juice	1 cup	1 cup	1 ½ cup	½ cup	1 cup	1 cup
Cheddar cheese, low-fat	-	-	¼ oz.	½ oz.	½ oz.	1 oz.

Directions: In a bowl, mix eggs, milk, and pepper. Boil asparagus for approximately 8 minutes. Set aside. Over medium-low heat, melt butter in frying pan. Add eggs, turn off heat, and cover with lid until eggs are cooked slightly. Add cheese and asparagus, then fold eggs over. Toast bagel. Place omelette on bagel.

DAY 2/MEAL 2

Banana Peach Shake

	1,600	1,800	2,000	2,200	2,400	2,600
Yogurt, plain, low-fat	¼ cup	⅓ cup	½ cup	½ cup	½ cup	⅔ cup
Banana	¾	¾	¾	1	1	1
Peach	¾	¾	¾	¾	1	1
Egg yolk	1	1	1	1	1	1
Vanilla high alpha whey isolate	1 (S)	1 ½ (S)	1 ½ (S)	1 ½ (S)	2 (S)	2 (S)
Almonds	¼ oz.	⅓ oz.	½ oz.	½ oz.	½ oz.	⅔ oz.

Directions: Place yogurt, banana, and peach in a blender and blend well. With blender on low speed, add egg yolk and protein. Continue blending for approximately 10 seconds. Eat nuts separately.

DAY 2/MEAL 3

Spinach Salad

	1,600	1,800	2,000	2,200	2,400	2,600
Spinach	1 ¾ cups	1 ¾ cups	2 cups	2 cups	2 cups	2 cups
Shrimp, large, raw	-	3	5	6	7	8
Pumpkin seeds, roasted	½ oz.	¾ oz.	⅔ oz.	¾ oz.	¾ oz.	1 oz.
Mozzarella, part skim	¼ cup	¼ cup	¼ cup	¼ cup	¼ cup	¼ cup
Mandarin oranges, canned in juice	¾ cup	1 cup	1 cup	1 cup	1 cup	1 ¼ cup
Egg	2 ½	2	2	2	2	2
Honey-miso dressing	1 ¼	1 ¼	1 ¼	1 ¼	1 ¾	2

Directions: Chop spinach and mozzarella cheese. Drain mandarin oranges. Mix spinach, carrots, mozzarella, and oranges together. Boil egg, let cool, discard yolk, then chop egg white and add to mixture. Toss with honey-miso dressing and add shrimp and pumpkin seeds. Mix well.

Miso dressing ingredients and instructions: Serves 7

In a bowl, mix all ingredients together.

Miso	3 tbsp.	Soy sauce	½ fluid oz.
Honey	2 tbsp.	Vinegar, cider	1 tbsp.
Mustard, Dijon	2 tsp.	Oil, olive	1 tsp.
Vegetable broth	2 tbsp.	Spice, ground ginger	1 tsp.
Green onions, chopped	1 tbsp.	Garlic clove, crushed	1

DAY 2/MEAL 4

Protein Boost

	1,600	1,800	2,000	2,200	2,400	2,600
Vanilla or chocolate high alpha whey isolate	1 (S)	1(HS)	1(HS)	1 ½ (S)	2 (S)	2 (S)
Soy milk	1 ¼ cup	1 ¼ cup	1 ½ cup	1 ½ cup	1 ½ cup	1 ½ cup
Almonds	8	11	13	13	14	15
Figs	3	3	3	4	4	5

Directions: Mix protein with soy milk in a shaker cup, or mix in blender on low speed for 5 to 10 seconds. Snack on almonds and figs.

DAY 2/MEAL 5

Fat Wars Chili

	1,600	1,800	2,000	2,200	2,400	2,600
Tomato paste	½ cup	½ cup	¾ cup	¾ cup	½ cup	½ cup
Tomato sauce	¼ cup	¼ cup	¼ cup	¼ cup	¼ cup	3 oz.
Garlic clove, fresh crushed	1	1	1	1	1	1 ¼
Kidney beans	¼ cup	¼ cup	3 oz.	3 oz.	3 oz.	½ cup
Ground beef, extra lean	1 oz.	1 ½ oz.	1 ½ oz.	2 oz.	2 oz.	2 oz.
Ground turkey	2 oz.	2 oz.	2 ½ oz.	2 ½ oz.	2 ½ oz.	3 oz.
Celery, chopped	2	2	2	2 ½	3	3
Carrots, chopped	1 oz.	1 oz.	1 oz.	1 ½ oz.	1 ½ oz.	1 ½ oz.
Onion, chopped	¼ cup	¼ cup	¼ cup	¼ cup	¼ cup	¼ cup

Directions: In skillet, cook ground beef and turkey on medium heat until brown. Drain excess fat. Drain kidney beans. Place all ingredients in a large pot. Bring to boil then simmer for 20 minutes.

DAY 3/MEAL 1

Organic Muesli

	1,600	1,800	2,000	2,200	2,400	2,600
Muesli	1 oz.	1 oz.	1 ¼ oz.	1 ¼ oz.	1 ⅓ oz.	1 ½ oz.
Yogurt, plain, low-fat	¼ cup	⅓ cup	¼ cup	½ cup	½ cup	⅔ cup
High alpha whey isolate	1 ½ (S)	1 ½ (S)	1 ½ (S)	1 ½ (S)	2 (S)	2 (S)
Almonds	⅓ oz.	½ oz.	½ oz.	½ oz.	½ oz.	½ oz.

Directions: Chop almonds into bite-size pieces, then mix all ingredients together.

DAY 3/MEAL 2

Hawaiian Pineapple Delight

	1,600	1,800	2,000	2,200	2,400	2,600
High alpha whey isolate	1 ½ (S)	1 ½ (S)	1 ½ (S)	1 ½ (S)	1 ½ (S)	2 (S)
Pineapple, diced	¼ cup	¼ cup	⅓ cup	⅓ cup	½ cup	½ cup
Pineapple juice	⅓ cup	⅓ cup	⅓ cup	⅓ cup	⅓ cup	½ cup
Yogurt, plain, low-fat	¼ cup	½ cup	½ cup	⅔ cup	¾ cup	¾ cup
Flaxseed, crushed	1 tsp.	1 tsp.	1 ¼ tsp.	1 ¼ tsp.	1 ⅓ tsp.	1 ⅓ tsp.

Directions: In blender, combine yogurt, diced pineapple, and juice. Blend well. Add protein and flaxseed. Blend for additional 10 seconds on low speed.

DAY 3/MEAL 3

Fruit Salad with Cottage Cheese

	1,600	1,800	2,000	2,200	2,400	2,600
Cottage cheese	¾ cup	⅔ cup	1 cup	1 cup	1 ¼ cup	1 ½ cup
Pineapple, canned in juice	⅛ cup	⅛ cup	⅛ cup	⅛ cup	¼ cup	¼ cup
Orange, fresh	½	⅔	¾	⅔	¾	¾
Peach, fresh	½	⅔	¾	⅔	¾	1
Strawberries, fresh	⅛ cup	⅛ cup	⅛ cup	⅛ cup	⅛ cup	¼ cup
Blackberries, fresh	⅛ cup	⅛ cup	⅛ cup	⅛ cup	⅛ cup	¼ cup
Cashews	⅔ oz.	¾ oz.	¾ oz.	1 oz.	1 oz.	1 oz.

Directions: Cut all fruit into bite-size pieces. Mix all fruit in a bowl with cottage cheese. Cashews are to be eaten separately.

DAY 3/MEAL 4

Holiday Shake

	1,600	1,800	2,000	2,200	2,400	2,600
Milk, 1%	¾ cup	1 cup	1 cup	1 ¼ cup	1 ¼ cup	1 ¼ cup
High alpha whey isolate	1 ½ (S)	1 ½ (S)	1 ½ (S)	1 ½ (S)	2 (S)	2 (S)
Honey	1 tbsp.	1 tbsp.	1 tbsp.	1 tbsp.	1 tbsp.	1 tbsp.
Ginger, ground	1 tsp.	1 tsp.	1 tsp.	1 tsp.	1 tsp.	1 tsp.
Nutmeg, ground	½ tsp.	½ tsp.	½ tsp.	¾ tsp.	¾ tsp.	¾ tsp.
Cinnamon, ground	½ tsp.	½ tsp.	½ tsp.	¾ tsp.	¾ tsp.	¾ tsp.
Almonds	½ oz.	½ oz.	¾ oz.	¾ oz.	⅛ oz.	1 oz.
Apple, fresh	¼ piece	¼ piece	¼ piece	⅓ piece	⅔ piece	½ piece

Directions: In a pot, warm milk, honey, ginger, nutmeg, and cinnamon. Pour into a shaker cup. Once cooled, add protein and shake until mixed. Almonds and apple are to be eaten separately.

DAY 3/MEAL 5

Salmon Delight

	1,600	1,800	2,000	2,200	2,400	2,600
Salmon, wild	3 ½ oz.	4 oz.	4 oz.	4 ½ oz.	5 oz.	5 ¼ oz.
Mushroom, shiitake, diced	¼ cup	¼ cup	⅓ cup	½ cup	½ cup	4 ½ oz.
Asparagus	½ cup	½ cup	4 ½ oz.	4 ½ oz.	5 oz.	¾ cup
Garlic clove, crushed	2	2	2 ½	3	3	3
Lemon	1	1 ¼	1 ¼	1 ¼	1 ⅓	1 ½
Wild rice	½ cup	½ cup	4 ½ oz.	4 ½ oz.	5 oz.	¾ cup

Directions: In pot, bring water (enough water to cover salmon) to boil. Add salmon and crushed garlic. Cover and simmer for 8 to 12 minutes or until fish flakes with fork. In a skillet, bring water (enough water to cover asparagus) to boil, add asparagus, and cook for 8 minutes. Cook rice according to package instructions, add raw mushrooms to rice, once water is boiling. Place asparagus over rice. Slice lemon and squeeze over salmon.

DAY 4/MEAL 1

Open-Faced Egg Muffin

	1,600	1,800	2,000	2,200	2,400	2,600
Egg, poached	2	2	2	2	2	2
Egg whites	1	1	1	1	2	2
English muffin, sourdough	½	½	½	½	½	¾
Butter	⅛ tbsp.	⅛ tbsp.	⅛ tbsp.	¼ tbsp.	¼ tbsp.	⅓ tbsp.
Salsa	⅓ cup	¼ cup	⅓ cup	¼ cup	¼ cup	¼ cup
Ham, lean baked	2 slices	3 slices	4 slices	4 slices	4 slices	4 slices
Grapefruit juice	1 cup	⅔ cup	¾ cup	1 cup	1 cup	1 cup

Directions: Poach eggs in boiling water. If adding egg whites, break whole egg into bowl, add egg whites to whole egg, then boil. Toast English muffin lightly. Heat ham slightly. Place English muffin on plate, butter, then cover with slices of ham, then poached eggs and the salsa. Grapefruit juice is to be consumed with meal.

DAY 4/MEAL 2

Carrot Top Shake

	1,600	1,800	2,000	2,200	2,400	2,600
Carrot juice	⅓ cup	½ cup	½ cup	½ cup	⅓ cup	½ cup
Orange, fresh, peeled	½	½	½	¾	1	1
Lemon juice	⅔ tbsp.	⅔ tbsp.	⅔ tbsp.	⅔ tbsp.	½ tbsp.	⅔ tbsp.
Flaxseed, crushed	1 tsp.	1 tsp.	1 ¼ tsp.	1 ¼ tsp.	1 ⅓ tsp.	1 ½ tsp.
Ginger, ground	¼ tsp.	¼ tsp.	¼ tsp.	¼ tsp.	¼ tsp.	¼ tsp.
Yogurt, plain, low-fat	¼ cup	⅓ cup	⅓ cup	½ cup	¾ cup	½ cup
High alpha whey isolate	1 ½ (S)	1 ½ (S)	1 ½ (S)	1 ½ (S)	1 ½ (S)	2 (S)

Directions: In blender, combine carrot juice, fresh orange, lemon juice, ginger, and yogurt. Blend well. Add protein and flaxseed to mixture and continue blending for 10 seconds on low speed.

DAY 4/MEAL 3

Roast Beef Sandwich

	1,600	1,800	2,000	2,200	2,400	2,600
Bread, 100% whole-wheat, stone-ground	2	2	2	2	2	2
Roast beef slices, deli, lean	2 oz.	2 ½	2 ½	3	3	3 ½
Monterey Jack cheese, light	⅓ oz.	⅓ oz.	¼ oz.	⅓ oz.	¾ oz.	1
Almond butter	⅔ tbsp.	⅔ tbsp.	1 tbsp.	1 tbsp.	1 tbsp.	1 tbsp.
Tomato	1 slice	2 slices	2 slices	3 slices	3 slices	3 slices
Parsley	½ tbsp.	½ tbsp.	½ tbsp.	½ tbsp.	⅓ tbsp.	½ tbsp.
Pickles, large, sliced	1 ¼	1 ¼	1 ½	2	2	2
Grapes	15	20	25	25	35	40

Directions: Toast bread lightly. Mix almond butter with parsley and spread over one side of the bread. Add roast beef, cheese, tomato, and sliced pickle. Grapes are to be eaten separately.

DAY 4/MEAL 4

Protein Rush

	1,600	1,800	2,000	2,200	2,400	2,600
Chocolate or vanilla high alpha whey isolate	1 ½ (S)	1 ½ (S)	2 (S)	2 (S)	2 ¼ (S)	2 ¼ (S)
Raisins, seedless	½ cup	¼ cup	¼ cup	½ cup	⅓ cup	⅓ cup
Almonds	¾ oz.	7/8 oz.	1 oz.	1 oz.	1 oz.	1 ¼ oz.
Peach, fresh	½	¼	½	¼	¾	¼

Directions: Mix protein in a shaker cup. Mix almonds and raisins together and consume. Eat peach separately.

DAY 4/MEAL 5

Mandarin/Chicken Salad

	1,600	1,800	2,000	2,200	2,400	2,600
Chicken breast, skinless	2 ½ oz.	2 ½ oz.	2 ¾ oz.	3 oz.	3 ½ oz.	4 oz.
Lettuce, mixed greens	2 cups	2 cups	2 cups	2 ¼ cup	2 ¼ cup	2 ½ cup
Mandarin oranges, canned in juice	1 cup	1 ¼ cup	1 ¼ cup	1 ⅓ cup	1 ½ cup	1 ⅔ cup
Pumpkin seeds	½ oz.	½ oz.	⅔ oz.	⅔ oz.	⅔ oz.	⅔ oz.
Balsamic Vinaigrette (Newman's Own)	¼ tbsp.	½ tbsp.	½ tbsp.	⅔ tbsp.	¾ tbsp.	1 tbsp.

Directions: Broil or roast chicken until cooked. Let cool, then chop up chicken. Drain mandarin oranges. Toss all ingredients together.

DAY 5/MEAL 1

Granola with Strawberries

	1,600	1,800	2,000	2,200	2,400	2,600
Granola, low-fat	¼ cup	¼ cup	¼ cup	¼ cup	¼ cup	½ cup
Yogurt, plain, low-fat	¼ cup	¼ cup	½ cup	⅔ cup	½ cup	½ cup
Vanilla or plain high alpha whey isolate	1 ½ (S)	1 ½ (S)	1 ½ (S)	1 ½ (S)	2 (S)	2 (S)
Strawberries	¼ cup	¼ cup	⅓ cup	½ cup	½ cup	½ cup
Flaxseed, crushed	¾ tsp.	1 tsp.	1 tsp.	1 ¼ tsp.	1 ¼ tsp.	1 ½ tsp.

Directions: Mix all ingredients in a bowl until desired consistency.

DAY 5/MEAL 2

Sweet and Sour Shake

	1,600	1,800	2,000	2,200	2,400	2,600
Strawberries, fresh	½ cup	½ cup	½ cup	½ cup	½ cup	½ cup
Pineapple, diced	¼ cup	⅓ cup	¼ cup	¼ cup	⅓ cup	½ cup
Grapefruit, whole, peeled	⅛	¼	¼	¼	¼	¼
Honey	¼ tbsp.	⅓ tbsp.	½ tbsp.	½ tbsp.	½ tbsp.	½ tbsp.
Yogurt, plain, low-fat	¼ cup	⅓ cup	½ cup	½ cup	½ cup	½ cup
Flaxseed, crushed	1 tsp.	1 tsp.	1 tsp.	1 ¼ tsp.	1 ⅓ tsp.	1 ½ tsp.
High alpha whey isolate	1 ½ (S)	1 ½ (S)	1 ½ (S)	1 ½ (S)	2 (S)	2 (S)

Directions: In blender, combine all ingredients except protein and flaxseed. Blend well, then add protein and flaxseed and blend for additional 10 seconds on low speed.

DAY 5/MEAL 3

Anytime Burrito

	1,600	1,800	2,000	2,200	2,400	2,600
Egg, whole	1	1	2	2	2	2
Egg whites	3	3	3	4	5	5
Tortilla, 100% whole-wheat	1	1	1	1	1	1
Salsa	¼ cup	¼ cup	⅓ cup	⅓ cup	½ cup	½ cup
Mozzarella cheese, part skim	⅛ cup	¼ cup	⅛ cup	⅛ cup	⅛ cup	¼ cup
Grapes	10	15	15	20	25	25

Directions: Slightly warm tortilla. Poach eggs as you like them. Place eggs and salsa on tortilla and cover with mozzarella. Fold tortilla up. Eat grapes separately. Remember: The softer the egg is poached, the messier the wrap will be.

DAY 5/MEAL 4

Blueberry Shake-It

	1,600	1,800	2,000	2,200	2,400	2,600
Vanilla or plain high alpha whey isolate	1 ½ (S)	2 (S)	2 (S)	2 (S)	2 ½ (S)	2 ⅓ (S)
Blueberries	½ cup	⅔ cup	⅓ cup	¾ cup	¾ cup	1 cup
Yogurt, plain, low-fat	⅔ cup	½ cup	¾ cup	¾ cup	¾ cup	¾ cup
Flaxseed oil	⅔ tbsp.	¾ tbsp.	¾ tbsp.	¾ tbsp.	1 tbsp.	1 tbsp.

Directions: Combine blueberries and yogurt and mix well in blender. Add protein and flaxseed oil and blend for approximately 10 seconds on low speed.

DAY 5/MEAL 5

Shrimp Stir-fry

	1,600	1,800	2,000	2,200	2,400	2,600
Shrimp, large	13	14	16	17	18	20
Broccoli, chopped	¼ cup	¼ cup	¼ cup	¼ cup	¼ cup	½ cup
Celery stick, chopped	1	2	3	3	3	3
Water chestnuts, sliced	⅛ cup	⅛ cup	¼ cup	¼ cup	¼ cup	¼ cup
Bean sprouts	¼ cup	¼ cup	¼ cup	¼ cup	¼ cup	¼ cup
Onion, slice, chopped	1	2	2	2	2 ½	3
Garlic clove	1	1	1	1	1	1 ½
Olive oil	⅔ tbsp.	¾ tbsp.	¾ tbsp.	1 tbsp.	1 tbsp.	1 ¼ tbsp.
Teriyaki sauce	1 oz.	1 oz.	1 ¼ oz.	1 ½ oz.	2 oz.	2 oz.
Wild rice	½ cup	¾ cup	¾ cup	¾ cup	¾ cup	¾ cup

Directions: Cook rice as per instructions on package. Heat skillet. Add olive oil. Crush garlic into the olive oil, then add broccoli, water chestnuts, onion, celery, bean sprouts, and shrimp. Stir-fry until everything is cooked, then add teriyaki sauce.

DAY 6/MEAL 1

Egg Breakfast

	1,600	1,800	2,000	2,200	2,400	2,600
Egg, whole	1	1	1	1	1	1
Egg white	2	3	3	3	4	5
Bread, oatmeal	1	1	1	2	2	2
Cheddar cheese, low-fat	1 oz.	1 ⅓ oz.	1 ½ oz.	1 ⅓ oz.	1 ½ oz.	1 ⅔ oz.
Butter	¼ tbsp.	⅓ tbsp.	½ tbsp.	½ tbsp.	⅔ tbsp.	½ tbsp.
Grapefruit (medium)	1	1	-	1	1	-
Grapefruit (large)	-	-	1	-	-	1

Directions: Lightly toast bread, then butter it. Poach the egg and egg white. Shred cheese. Place grated cheese and poached eggs on the toast. The warmth of the toast and the eggs will slightly melt the cheese. Grapefruit is to be eaten separately.

DAY 6/MEAL 2

Orchard Blend

	1,600	1,800	2,000	2,200	2,400	2,600
Vanilla high alpha whey isolate	2 (S)	2 (S)	2 ½ (S)	2 ½ (S)	2 ⅓ (S)	2 ½ (S)
Peach	½	¾	¾	1	1 ¼	1
Orange	¾	¾	¾	1	1 ¼	1
Banana	½	¾	¾	¾	¾	1
Water	½ cup	½ cup	½ cup	½ cup	½ cup	½ cup
Flaxseed oil	¾ tbsp.	¾ tbsp.	1 tbsp.	1 tbsp.	1 tbsp.	1 ¼ tbsp.

Directions: Mix peach, orange, and banana in blender with water. Blend well. Add protein and flaxseed oil, continue blending for approximately 10 seconds on low speed.

DAY 6/MEAL 3

Mexican Marvel

	1,600	1,800	2,000	2,200	2,400	2,600
Tortilla, whole-wheat	1	1	1	1	1	1
Ground turkey, lean	2 ½ oz.	3 oz.	3 oz.	3 ½ oz.	4 oz.	4 ½ oz.
Corn kernels	-	⅒ cup	¼ cup	⅓ cup	½ cup	½ cup
Taco seasoning	1	1	1	1	1 ¼	1 ⅓
Water	1 tsp.	1 tsp.	1 tsp.	1 tsp.	1 tsp.	1 tsp.
Cheddar cheese, low-fat	1 oz.	1 oz.	1 ¼ oz.	1 ¼ oz.	1 ⅓ oz.	1 ½ oz.
Salsa	½ oz.	½ oz.	⅔ oz.	⅔ oz.	¾ oz.	1 oz.
Apple	⅓	⅓	⅓	½	⅓	½

Directions: Cook ground turkey in skillet on low heat. Once browned, drain and add corn kernels and taco seasoning with water. Heat tortilla in oven on low. Place ground turkey mixture in center of tortilla, then cover with Cheddar cheese and salsa. Fold tortilla up like a fajita. Eat apple separately.

DAY 6/MEAL 4

Frozen Colada

	1,600	1,800	2,000	2,200	2,400	2,600
Pineapple, diced	½ cup	½ cup	½ cup	½ cup	½ cup	⅔ cup
Pineapple juice	⅛ cup	¼ cup	¼ cup	¼ cup	⅓ cup	⅓ cup
Frozen yogurt, vanilla	¼ cup	¼ cup	⅓ cup	⅓ cup	⅓ cup	⅓ cup
Water	½ cup	½ cup	½ cup	½ cup	½ cup	½ cup
Vanilla high alpha whey isolate	1 ½ (S)	1 ½ (S)	2 (S)	2 (S)	2 (S)	2 ½ (S)
Flaxseed, crushed	¾ tsp.	1 tsp.	1 tsp.	1 ¼ tsp.	1 ⅓ tsp.	1 ⅓ tsp.

Directions: In blender, combine pineapple juice and fruit with frozen yogurt and water. Blend well, add protein and flaxseed and blend for additional 10 seconds on low speed.

DAY 6/MEAL 5

A Real Steak Dinner

	1,600	1,800	2,000	2,200	2,400	2,600
Steak, lean sirloin	3 oz.	3 ½ oz.	4 oz.	4 oz.	4 oz.	5 oz.
Mushrooms, shiitake	⅓ cup	½ cup	⅔ cup	1 cup	1 ¼ cup	1 cup
Garlic clove, crushed	1	1	1	1 ½	1 ½	1 ½
Butter	½ tbsp.	½ tbsp.	½ tbsp.	⅔ tbsp.	⅔ tbsp.	¾ tbsp.
Asparagus	2	3	2	3	3	3
Red wine	3 oz.	3 oz.	3 oz.	3 oz.	3 oz.	4 oz.

Directions: Melt half the butter in a skillet on medium heat and cook steak until done to your liking. Place the rest of the butter in a skillet with garlic and sliced mushrooms. Cook on medium heat for approximately 8 minutes. Place asparagus in boiling water and cook for approximately 8 minutes. Enjoy the wine with your dinner.

DAY 7/MEAL 1

Berry Cottage Cheese

	1,600	1,800	2,000	2,200	2,400	2,600
Cottage cheese, 1%	⅔ cup	¾ cup	1 cup	1 cup	1 cup	1 ¼ cup
Blueberries	½ cup	½ cup	¾ cup	¾ cup	¾ cup	1 cup
Blackberries	¼ cup	¼ cup	¼ cup	¼ cup	¼ cup	¼ cup
Strawberries	¼ cup	¼ cup	⅛ cup	¼ cup	¼ cup	¼ cup
Flaxseed (crushed)	1 tsp.	1 tsp.	1 tsp.	1 ¼ tsp.	1 ½ tsp.	1 ½ tsp.

Directions: Stir flaxseed into cottage cheese, then add berries.

DAY 7/MEAL 2

Protein Punch

	1,600	1,800	2,000	2,200	2,400	2,600
Vanilla or chocolate high alpha whey isolate	2 (S)	2 (S)	2 ½ (S)	2 ⅓ (S)	2 ½ (S)	2 ¼ (S)
Flaxseed oil	¾ tbsp.	¾ tbsp.	1 tbsp.	1 tbsp.	1 tbsp.	1 ¼ tbsp.
Figs	1	2	2	2 ½	3	3
Apple (medium)	1	1	1	1	1	1 ¼

Directions: In a shaker cup, mix protein and flaxseed with water and shake. Figs and apple are to be eaten separately.

DAY 7/MEAL 3

Broccoli Soup and Chicken Sandwich

	1,600	1,800	2,000	2,200	2,400	2,600
Broccoli pieces	½ cup	½ cup	¾ cup	¾ cup	1 cup	1 cup
Vegetable cube	¾	1	1 ¼	1 ½	1 ½	2
Lemon juice	½ tbsp.	½ tbsp.	⅔ tbsp.	¾ tbsp.	1 tbsp.	1 tbsp.
Pepper	1 tsp.	1 tsp.	1 tsp.	1 tsp.	1 tsp.	1 ¼ tsp.
Pumpernickel bread	1	1	1	1	1	1
Chicken breast, lean, cooked	3 slices	4 slices	4 slices	4 ½ slices	5 slices	5 ½ slices
Mayonnaise	½ tbsp.	⅔ tbsp.	¾ tbsp.	¾ tbsp.	¾ tbsp.	1 tbsp.
Celery stalk	1	1	1 ¼	1 ½	1 ⅔	2
Tomato slices	1	2	3	4	4	3

Directions: Bring 1 ½ cups of water to boil. Add vegetable cube and broccoli and cook for approximately 10 minutes. Pour half the liquid into the blender and blend for approximately 30 seconds. Return blended liquid to soup and add lemon juice and pepper. Cut chicken into small chunks, dice celery, and mix both with mayonnaise. Place mixture on pumpernickel bread and cover with tomato slices.

DAY 7/MEAL 4

Yogurt Delight

	1,600	1,800	2,000	2,200	2,400	2,600
Yogurt, plain	1 cup	1 ¼ cup	1 ¼ cup	1 ¼ cup	1 ⅓ cup	1 ⅓ cup
Vanilla high alpha whey isolate	1 ½ (S)	1 ½ (S)	1 ½ (S)	2 (S)	2 (S)	2 ½ (S)
Apple	⅓	½	½	½	½	½
Pear	½	½	½	½	¾	1
Water	½ cup	½ cup	½ cup	½ cup	½ cup	½ cup
Flaxseed oil	¼ tbsp.	¼ tbsp.	1 tsp.	1 tsp.	½ tbsp.	½ tbsp.

Directions: Core apple and pear, but do not remove skin. In blender, mix yogurt, apple, and pear with water. Add proteins and flaxseed oil and blend for additional 10 seconds.

DAY 7/MEAL 5

Tuna with Greek Salad

	1,600	1,800	2,000	2,200	2,400	2,600
Tuna (bluefin)	3 oz.	3 oz.	4 oz.	4 oz.	4 ¼ oz.	4 ½ oz.
Green onion, chopped	½ tbsp.	½ tbsp.	⅔ tbsp.	¾ tbsp.	1 tbsp.	1 tbsp.
Wild rice	½ cup	¾ cup	¾ cup	⅔ cup	¾ cup	⅔ cup
Olive oil	½ tbsp.	½ tbsp.	⅔ tbsp.	⅔ tbsp.	⅔ tbsp.	¾ tbsp.
Cucumber, chopped	½ cup	½ cup	½ cup	¾ cup	¾ cup	¾ cup
Tomato	⅓	½	½	⅔	¾	¾
Bell peppers	½	½	½	⅔	¾	¾
Onion	¼ cup	¼ cup	¼ cup	¼ cup	½ cup	½ cup
Oregano	1 tsp.	1 tsp.	1 tsp.	1 tsp.	1 tsp.	1 tsp.
Lemon	½	½	⅔	¾	1	1

Directions: Bring water (enough to cover tuna) to a boil. Add tuna and cook for 8 to 10 minutes. Cook wild rice as per package instructions. Add green onions once water for rice has come to a boil.. Chop cucumber, tomato, bell peppers, and onion. Toss vegetables with olive oil and oregano.

DAY 8/MEAL 1

Muesli Delight

	1,600	1,800	2,000	2,200	2,400	2,600
Muesli (organic)	1 oz.	1 ¼ oz.	1 ¼ oz.	1 ½ oz.	1 ½ oz.	1 ½ oz.
Milk, 1%	¼ cup	¼ cup	⅓ cup	⅓ cup	½ cup	¾ cup
High alpha whey isolate	1 ½ (S)	1 ½ (S)	1 ½ (S)	2 (S)	2 (S)	2 (S)
Flaxseed oil	½ tbsp.	½ tbsp.	2 tsp.	2 tsp.	2 tsp.	2 ½ tsp.

Directions: Place all ingredients in a bowl. Mix until desired consistency.

DAY 8/MEAL 2

Really Good 4U Cheese Whiz

	1,600	1,800	2,000	2,200	2,400	2,600
High alpha whey isolate	1 (S)	1 (S)	1 ½ (S)	1 ½ (S)	1 ½ (S)	2 (S)
Celery stick	5	5 ½	6	6	6	7
Cream cheese, light	1 ½ oz.	1 ¾ oz.	1 ¾ oz.	2 oz.	2 ¼ oz.	2 ½ oz.
Green onion, chopped	¼ cup	½ cup	¾ oz.	1 cup	1 cup	1 cup
Artichoke, canned whole (chopped)	3	3 ½	4	4	4	4 ½
Paprika	1 tsp.	1 ¼ tsp.	1 ⅓ tsp.	1 ⅓ tsp.	1 ⅓ tsp.	1 ½ tsp.
Garlic clove, crushed	1	1 ¼	1 ⅓	1 ⅓	1 ⅓	1 ½
Spinach, chopped finely	¼ cup	¼ cup	3 oz.	3 oz.	3 oz.	3 oz.

Directions: In a shaker cup, mix proteins with water. In a bowl, combine all ingredients except celery and paprika. Mix until desired consistency. Spread mixture on celery sticks and sprinkle with paprika

DAY 8/MEAL 3

Tuna Sandwich

	1,600	1,800	2,000	2,200	2,400	2,600
Tuna, solid white (in water)	3 oz.	3.5 oz.	4 oz.	4 ¼ oz.	4 ½ oz.	5 oz.
Pita bread (oat-bran)	½ piece	½ piece	½ piece	¾ piece	1 piece	1 piece
Mayonnaise (organic)	2 tsp.	2 tsp.	1 tbsp.	1 tbsp.	1 tbsp.	1 tbsp.
Tomato	½	½	½	½	½	1
Cucumber	¼ cup	¼ cup	¼ cup	¼ cup	¼ cup	¼ cup
Apple	¾	1	1	1	1	1

Directions: Chop or dice tomato and cucumber. Combine tuna, tomato, cucumber, and mayonnaise. Place in pita shell. Eat apple separately.

DAY 8/MEAL 4

Strawberry/Rhubarb Shake

	1,600	1,800	2,000	2,200	2,400	2,600
Water	½ cup	½ cup	½ cup	½ cup	½ cup	½ cup
High alpha whey isolate	2 (S)	2 (S)	2 (S)	2 ¼ (S)	2 ½ (S)	2 ½ (S)
Strawberries	¾ cup	1 cup	1 ¼ cup	1 ¼ cup	1 ½ cup	1 ¾ cup
Rhubarb	¾ cup	1 cup	1 ¼ cup	1 ¼ cup	1 ½ cup	1 ¾ cup
Honey (unpasteurized)	1 tbsp.	1 tbsp.	1 ¼ tbsp.	1 ¼ tbsp.	1 ¼ tbsp.	4 tsp.
Flaxseed oil	¾ tbsp.	1 tbsp.	1 tbsp.	1 ¼ tbsp.	1 ¼ tbsp.	4 tsp.

Directions: Using water as the base, add fruit and honey to blender, then mix on medium for 10 to 15 seconds. Turn blender to low and add protein and flaxseed oil. Blend for additional 10 seconds.

DAY 8/MEAL 5

Lamb with Wild Rice

	1,600	1,800	2,000	2,200	2,400	2,600
Lamb, cubed	2 ½ oz.	3 oz.	3 oz.	3 ½ oz.	3 ½ oz.	4 oz.
Butter	¼ tbsp.	¼ tbsp.	¼ tbsp.	¼ tbsp.	¼ tbsp.	¼ tbsp.
Thyme, fresh	½ tsp.	½ tsp.	½ tsp.	½ tsp.	⅓ tsp.	⅓ tsp.
Pepper	¼ tsp.	¼ tsp.	¼ tsp.	⅓ tsp.	¼ tsp.	¼ tsp.
Celery, chopped	1 piece	1 piece	1 piece	1 piece	1 piece	1 piece
Carrots, chopped	⅛ cup	⅛ cup	¼ cup	¼ cup	⅛ cup	⅛ cup
Green onion	1 tbsp.	1 tbsp.	1 tbsp.	1 tbsp.	1 tbsp.	1 tbsp.
Wild rice	¼ cup	¼ cup	⅓ cup	⅓ cup	½ cup	½ cup
Chicken broth	¼ cup	¼ cup	¼ cup	¼ cup	¼ cup	¼ cup
Garlic clove, crushed	1	1	1	1	1	1
Butter	½ tbsp.	½ tbsp.	½ tbsp.	⅔ tbsp.	¾ tbsp.	¾ tbsp.
Red wine	2 oz.	3 oz.	3 oz.	3 oz.	3 oz.	4 oz.

Directions: Remove broiler pan from oven, turn oven to broil. Cut lamb into cubes and place on skewers. Prepare rice as per directions on package, using chicken broth as well as water. Chop celery, carrots, pepper, and green onion into small pieces. Add vegetables and crushed garlic to rice when water comes to a boil. Vegetables will cook with rice. Melt butter, mix with thyme, and brush over lamb. Place skewers on unheated rack of broiler pan. Broil 3 inches from heat for 6 to 8 minutes for medium-cooked lamb, turning skewers often. Enjoy wine with meal.

DAY 9/MEAL 1

Peanut Butter and Banana

	1,600	1,800	2,000	2,200	2,400	2,600
Sprouted grain bread	1	1	1	1	1	1
Peanut butter (organic)	1 tbsp.	1 ¼ tbsp.	1 ⅓ tbsp.	1 ½ tbsp.	1 ⅔ tbsp.	1 ¾ tbsp.
Banana	½	½	¾	1	1	1 ¼
Vanilla or chocolate high alpha whey isolate	1 ½ (S)	1 ½ (S)	1 ½ (S)	1 ½ (S)	2 (S)	2 (S)

Directions: Toast bread. Spread peanut butter on toast. Slice banana and place on top of peanut butter. Mix protein with water.

DAY 9/MEAL 2

Phyto Nutrient Delight

	1,600	1,800	2,000	2,200	2,400	2,600
transform+™	2½ (S)	2½ (S)	2½ (S)	2 ⅓ (S)	2½ (S)	2½ (S)
Organic apple juice	¼ cup	¼ cup	⅓ cup	⅓ cup	½ cup	½ cup
Water	¾ cup	¾ cup	¾ cup	¾ cup	¾ cup	¾ cup
Mixed berries	5 oz.	½ cup	½ cup	5 oz.	5 oz.	½ cup
Banana	⅓	⅓	½	⅓	⅓	½
Flaxseed, crushed	¾ tsp.	1 tsp.	1 tsp.	1 ⅓ tsp.	1 ⅓ tsp.	1 ½ tsp.

Directions: Place ½ cup water in a blender with apple juice. Add mixed berries and banana and blend for 10 seconds on medium or high. Turn blender speed to low and add flaxseed and transform+. Blend for another 5 to 10 seconds. Add water if drink is too thick.

DAY 9/MEAL 3

Super Chicken Soup

	1,600	1,800	2,000	2,200	2,400	2,600
Chicken broth	1 cup	1 cup	1 cup	1 cup	1 cup	1 cup
Water	1 cup	1 cup	1 cup	1 cup	1 cup	1 cup
Chicken, cooked and diced	⅓ cup	½ cup	½ cup	½ cup	⅔ cup	⅔ cup
Egg noodles, fine	1 ¾ oz.	1 ¾ oz.	2 oz.	2 oz.	2 oz.	2 ¼ oz.
Leeks, raw, chopped	¼ cup	¼ cup	¼ cup	¼ cup	¼ cup	¼ cup
Butter	⅓ tbsp.	⅓ tbsp.	⅓ tbsp.	½ tbsp.	½ tbsp.	½ tbsp.

Directions: Cook egg noodles according to directions on package. Sauté leeks in butter for 5 minutes over medium-low heat. Add diced chicken. Add chicken broth and water. Bring to a boil, then turn heat to low, add cooked egg noodles, and let soup simmer for 5 minutes.

DAY 9/MEAL 4

Kiwi/Banana Rama

	1,600	1,800	2,000	2,200	2,400	2,600
Vanilla high alpha whey isolate	2 (S)	2 ½ (S)	2 ¼ (S)	2 ⅓ (S)	2 ⅓ (S)	2 ½ (S)
Kiwi	⅔	¾	1	1	1 ¼	1 ⅓
Banana	1	1	1	1 ¼	1 ¼	1 ⅓
Flaxseed oil	¾ tbsp.	¾ tbsp.	1 tbsp.	1 tbsp.	1 ¼ tbsp.	1⅓ tbsp.

Directions: In blender, combine kiwi, banana and water, blend well. Add protein and flaxseed and blend for additional 10 seconds.

DAY 9/MEAL 5

Scallop Jambalaya

	1,600	1,800	2,000	2,200	2,400	2,600
Scallops	4 oz.	4 ½ oz.	5 oz.	5 oz.	5 oz.	5 ½ oz.

Celery stalk	1	1 ¼	2	2 ½	3	3 ½
Onion slice	1	1 ¼	2	2 ½	3	3 ½
Pepper, green, red, or orange	¼	⅓	½	⅔	¾	1
Butter	⅔ tbsp.	¾ tbsp.	¾ tbsp.	1 tbsp.	1 tbsp.	1 tbsp.
Canned tomatoes with liquid	¼ cup	¼ cup	⅓ cup	½ cup	½ cup	⅔ cup
Chicken broth	½ cup	⅔ cup	¾ cup	1 cup	1 cup	1 ¼ cup
Brown rice, long-grain	½ cup	½ cup	½ cup	½ cup	⅔ cup	¾ cup
Hot pepper sauce	¾ tsp.	1 tsp.	1 ¼ tsp.	1 ⅓ tsp.	1 ½ tsp.	1 ½ tsp.
Garlic clove	1	1	1	1	2	2
Basil	¾ tsp.	1 tsp.	1 ¼ tsp.	1 ⅓ tsp.	1 ½ tsp.	1 ½ tsp.

Directions: Chop celery, onion, and pepper into bite-size pieces. In skillet, melt butter and cook celery, onion, and pepper. Add chicken broth, canned tomatoes and liquid, rice, basil, hot pepper sauce, and garlic. Cover and cook for approximately 20 minutes or until rice is cooked. Meanwhile, stir-fry scallops on medium heat for approximately 9 minutes. Once rice is cooked, add scallops.

DAY 10/MEAL 1

Spinach and Feta Eggs

	1,600	1,800	2,000	2,200	2,400	2,600
Eggs, whole	1	1	2	1	1	2
Egg white	2	3	2	4	4	3
Feta cheese	½ oz.	⅔ oz.	⅓ oz.	1 oz.	1 ¼ oz.	1 oz.
Spinach	¼ cup	½ cup	½ cup	¾ cup	½ cup	½ cup
Red onion	¼ cup	¼ cup	¼ cup	¼ cup	¼ cup	¼ cup
16-grain bread, slice	1	1	1	1	1	1
Grapefruit	½	¾	1	1	1 ¼	1 ½

Directions: Boil spinach for 8 minutes. Poach egg and egg white. Toast bread. Place boiled spinach and red onion on toast. Sprinkle with feta cheese and place poached eggs on top. Eat grapefruit separately.

DAY 10/MEAL 2

Protein Dream

	1,600	1,800	2,000	2,200	2,400	2,600
High alpha whey isolate	2 (S)	2 (S)	2 ¼ (S)	2 ⅓ (S)	2 ½ (S)	2 ½ (S)
Vanilla Rice Dream	1 cup	1 ¼ cup	1 ⅓ cup	1 ½ cup	1 ½ cup	1 ¾ cup
Flaxseed oil	2 tsp.	2 tsp.	2 tsp.	2 tsp.	1 tbsp.	1 tbsp.

Directions: Pour Rice Dream into a shaker cup. Add protein and flaxseed oil and shake vigorously for 10 seconds.

DAY 10/MEAL 3

You Betcha—It's a Pizza!

	1,600	1,800	2,000	2,200	2,400	2,600
Pita, whole-wheat	1	1	1	1	1	1
Tomato sauce	⅛ cup	⅛ cup	⅛ cup	⅛ cup	⅛ cup	⅛ cup
Cheddar cheese	¾ oz.	1 oz.	½ oz.	¾ oz.	⅔ oz.	¾ oz.
Mozzarella cheese	½ oz.	½ oz.	1 oz.	½ oz.	1 oz.	½ oz.
Feta cheese	¼ oz.	¼ oz.	¾ oz.	¾ oz.	1 oz.	1 oz.
Shrimp	4 ½	5	7	7	7	8
Artichoke, chopped	3 ½	4	5	6	6	7

Directions: Top pita with tomato sauce, shrimp, chopped artichoke, feta, mozzarella, and Cheddar. Bake in oven at 350°F for 15 minutes or until cheese is fully melted.

DAY 10/MEAL 4

Grapefruity

	1,600	1,800	2,000	2,200	2,400	2,600
Cottage cheese, 1%	⅔ cup	¾ cup	¾ cup	¾ cup	1 cup	1 cup
Grapefruit	1	1	½	1	1	1
Apple	-	-	½	⅓	¼	½
Flaxseed, crushed	1 tsp.	1 tsp.	1 ¼ tsp.	1 ⅓ tsp.	1 ½ tsp.	1 ½ tsp.

Directions: Cut grapefruit and apple into bite-size pieces. Mix flaxseed into cottage cheese and add fruit.

DAY 10/MEAL 5

Steak Kabob

	1,600	1,800	2,000	2,200	2,400	2,600
Beef, lean (cubed)	3 oz.	3 ½ oz.	3 ½ oz.	3 ½ oz.	4 oz.	4 oz.
Zucchini, sliced	¼ cup	⅛ cup	¼ cup	¼ cup	¼ cup	½ cup
Onion slice	2	1 ½	2	2	2	4
Tomato, cherry	¼	¼	¼	¼	¼	⅓
Lettuce, mixed greens	¼ cup	¼ cup	¼ cup	¼ cup	¼ cup	¼ cup
Oil and Vinegar, Newman's Own	⅓ tbsp.	½ tbsp.	½ tbsp.	⅔ tbsp.	⅔ tbsp.	⅔ tbsp.
Wild rice	¼ cup	⅓ cup	½ cup	½ cup	½ cup	½ cup
Apple	½	½	½	½	⅔	¾
Orange	½	½	½	⅔	⅔	⅔

Directions: In boiling water, cook zucchini for 3 minutes. On skewer, place beef, zucchini, and onion. Use half the oil and vinegar to baste skewered vegetables. Place on unheated rack of broiler pan. Broil for 5 to 6 minutes (or to desired doneness) 3 inches from heat. Add tomatoes to skewer for last 3 minutes. In bowl, mix lettuce and remaining dressing. Cook wild rice as per package instructions. Apple and orange are to be cut and eaten as dessert.

DAY 11/MEAL 1

Poached Eggs 'n' Cheese

	1,600	1,800	2,000	2,200	2,400	2,600
Egg	1	1 ¼	1 ⅓	1 ½	1 ½	2
Cheddar cheese, low-fat	1 ½ oz.	1 ½ oz.	1 ¾ oz.	2 ¼ oz.	2 ¼ oz.	2 ½ oz.
Oat bran (Red Mill)	¼ cup	3 oz.	½ cup	½ cup	5 oz.	5 oz.
Rice Dream	⅓ cup	⅓ cup	⅓ cup	⅓ cup	⅓ cup	⅓ cup

Directions: Poach egg. (For less than whole servings of eggs, please poach first, then cut to alloted size.) Top egg with Cheddar cheese, and let the heat of the egg melt the cheese. Add oat bran to boiling water and cover. Turn heat off and let sit for 10 minutes. Add Rice Dream to oat bran.

DAY 11/MEAL 2

Berry Orange

	1,600	1,800	2,000	2,200	2,400	2,600
Vanilla high alpha whey isolate	2 (S)	2 ½ (S)	2 ¼ (S)	2 ⅓ (S)	2 ½ (S)	2 ½ (S)
Strawberries	¼ cup	½ cup	½ cup	⅔ cup	¾ cup	¾ cup
Orange, medium	½	¾	⅓	½	½	½
Water	½ cup	½ cup	½ cup	½ cup	½ cup	½ cup
Flaxseed oil	¾ tbsp.	1 tbsp.	1 tbsp.	1 tbsp.	1 ¼ tbsp.	1 ¼ tbsp.
Figs, raw	2	2	3	3	3	4

Directions: In blender, mix strawberries and orange with ½ cup water. Blend well. Add protein and flaxseed and blend an additional 10 seconds on low. Figs are to be eaten separately.

DAY 11/MEAL 3

Egg Salad Sandwich

	1,600	1,800	2,000	2,200	2,400	2,600
Bread, 16-grain, slice	1	1	1	2	2	2
Egg white	3	4	4	4	5	6
Egg, whole (medium)	1	1	1	1	1	1
Mayonnaise, organic	½ tbsp.	½ tbsp.	⅔ tbsp.	⅔ tbsp.	¾ tbsp.	1 tbsp.
Celery stalk	1	2	2	2	2	2
Cucumber slices	⅛ cup	⅛ cup	¼ cup	¼ cup	¼ cup	⅓ cup
Dijon mustard	¼ tsp.	¼ tsp.	¼ tsp.	¼ tsp.	¼ tsp.	¼ tsp.
Tomato juice	1 cup	1 ¼ cup	1 ½ cup	¾ cup	¾ cup	1 cup

Directions: Boil eggs. Remove yolks from those eggs that should contain white only. Chop eggs and celery, then mix with mayonnaise and Dijon mustard. Layer cucumbers on bread, then top with egg mixture.

DAY 11/MEAL 4

Chocolate Dreams

	1,600	1,800	2,000	2,200	2,400	2,600
Chocolate high alpha whey isolate	2 (S)	2 (S)	2 ½ (S)	2 ¼ (S)	2 ½ (S)	2 ½ (S)
Rice Dream (chocolate)	⅔ cup	⅔ cup	¾ cup	1 cup	1 cup	1 cup
Flaxseed oil	⅔ tbsp.	¾ tbsp.	¾ tbsp.	1 tbsp.	1 tbsp.	1 tbsp.
Banana	½	⅔	¾	½	½	1

Directions: In a shaker cup, mix protein, Rice Dream, and flaxseed oil. Eat banana separately.

DAY 11/MEAL 5

Salmon and Stuffed Pepper

	1,600	1,800	2,000	2,200	2,400	2,600
Salmon, wild coho	3 oz.	3 oz.	3 ½ oz.	4 oz.	4 ½ oz.	4 ¾ oz.
Pepper (green or red)	1	1	1	1	1	1
Wild rice	½ cup	⅔ cup	¾ cup	¾ cup	¾ cup	1 cup
Celery	1	1	1	2	2	2
Onion, slice	1	1	1	3	3	3
Chicken broth	½ cup	⅔ cup	⅔ cup	¾ cup	¾ cup	¾ cup
Butter	½ tbsp.	½ tbsp.	½ tbsp.	½ tbsp.	½ tbsp.	½ tbsp.
Lemon	½	½	½	½	½	½
Garlic clove	1	1	1	1	1	1

Directions: Boil salmon for 8 minutes (add in crushed garlic). Cook rice as per directions on package, including allotted butter serving above, and use chicken broth instead of water. If there is not enough chicken broth, supplement with water. Chop celery and onion and add to rice when liquid comes to a boil. The vegetables will cook with the rice. Cut top off pepper and remove seeds and core. Place pepper in oven for 3 minutes at 350°F. Scoop cooked rice mixture into pepper. Wrap pepper in tin foil and bake in oven for additional 8 minutes. Lemon is to be used as a garnish for the salmon.

DAY 12/MEAL 1

7-Grain Hot Cereal

	1,600	1,800	2,000	2,200	2,400	2,600
Water	2 cups	2 cups	2 cups	2 ½ (S)	2 ½ (S)	2 cups
7-Grain Hot Cereal (Red Mill)	4 tbsp.	5 tbsp.	5 tbsp.	5 tbsp.	6 tbsp.	6 tbsp.
High alpha whey isolate	1 ½ (S)	2 (S)	2 (S)	2 (HS)	2 (HS)	2 ⅓ (S)
Banana (sliced)	⅓	⅓	⅓	½	½	½
Flaxseed oil	2 tsp.	2 tsp.	1 tbsp.	1 tbsp.	1 tbsp.	1 ¼ tbsp.

Directions: Boil water. Add allotted measurement of cereal to the boiling water and reduce heat to low. Cook for 10 minutes, stirring occasionally. When cereal is ready, let stand until warm, then mix in other ingredients.

DAY 12/MEAL 2

Frozen Blue

	1,600	1,800	2,000	2,200	2,400	2,600
Frozen yogurt, plain	½ cup	½ cup	½ cup	⅔ cup	⅔ cup	⅔ cup
Blueberries	½ cup	½ cup	¾ cup	¾ cup	¾ cup	¾ cup
Peach	½	½	½	⅓	1	¾
Water	¼ cup	¼ cup	¼ cup	¼ cup	¼ cup	¼ cup
Vanilla high alpha whey isolate	1 ½ (S)	2 (S)	2 (S)	2 ¼ (S)	2 ⅓ (S)	2 ⅓ (S)
Flaxseed oil	½ tbsp.	⅔ tbsp.	¾ tbsp.	¾ tbsp.	¾ tbsp.	1 tbsp.

Directions: In blender, combine yogurt, blueberries, peach, and water. Blend well. Add protein and flaxseed oil and blend on low for additional 10 seconds.

DAY 12/MEAL 3

Shrimp Salad

	1,600	1,800	2,000	2,200	2,400	2,600
Shrimp	16	19	19	22	22	25
Lettuce, mixed greens	1 cup	1 cup	1 ¼ cup	1 ½ cup	1 ¾ cup	2 cups
Onion, slices	3	3	4	4	5	6
Mushroom, shiitake	¾ cup	¾ cup	1 cup	1 cup	1 cup	1 cup
Cheese, mozzarella, shredded	-	-	-	-	½ oz.	½ oz.
Balsamic Vinaigrette, Newman's Own	¾ tbsp.	¾ tbsp.	1 tbsp.	1 tbsp.	1 ¼ tbsp.	1 ⅓ tbsp.
Cashews	½ oz.	⅔ oz.	⅔ oz.	¾ oz.	¾ oz.	¾ oz.
Water chestnuts	½ cup	⅓ cup	⅓ cup	⅓ cup	½ cup	½ cup

Directions: Chop onions, mushrooms, water chestnuts, and finely chop cashews into bite-size pieces. Mix all ingredients together (except dressing and cheese). Toss with dressing, and add cheese.

DAY 12/MEAL 4

Green Beret

	1,600	1,800	2,000	2,200	2,400	2,600
Strawberry transform+	2 (S)	2 ½ (S)	2 ½ (S)	2 ½ (S)	2 ½ (S)	2 ½ (S)
Flaxseed oil	½ tbsp.	½ tbsp.	⅔ tbsp.	⅔ tbsp.	⅔ tbsp.	⅔ tbsp.
Melon	¾ cup	1 cup	1 cup	1 cup	1 cup	1 cup
Kiwi, medium	1	1	1	1 ½	1 ½	1 ½
Yogurt, plain	⅓ cup	⅓ cup	½ cup	½ cup	¾ cup	1 cup
Water	½ cup	½ cup	½ cup	½ cup	½ cup	½ cup

Directions: In blender, place melon, kiwi, and yogurt with water. Blend well. Add transform+ and flaxseed oil and blend on low for additional 10 seconds.

DAY 12/MEAL 5

I Yam a Steak

	1,600	1,800	2,000	2,200	2,400	2,600
Steak, lean sirloin	2 ½ oz.	3 oz.	3 ¼ oz.	3 ½ oz.	4 oz.	4 ½ oz.
Teriyaki sauce	2 tbsp.	2 tbsp.	2 tbsp.	2 tbsp.	2 tbsp.	2 tbsp.
Yam	½ cup	⅔ cup	¾ cup	¾ cup	¾ cup	¾ cup
Carrots	½ cup	½ cup	½ cup	¾ cup	¾ cup	¾ cup
Butter	⅓ tbsp.	⅓ tbsp.	⅓ tbsp.	⅓ tbsp.	⅓ oz.	½ oz.

Directions: Marinate steak in teriyaki sauce for 10 minutes, then flip the steak over and marinate the other side for additional 10 minutes. Cook steak with remaining sauce on medium heat until done. In boiling water, cook yam 15 to 20 minutes. Drain well. Steam carrots for 8 minutes on top of stove. Mash cooked vegetables together and add butter.

DAY 13/MEAL 1

Yogurt Fruit Salad

	1,600	1,800	2,000	2,200	2,400	2,600
Vanilla high alpha whey isolate	1 (S)	1 ½ (S)	1 ½ (S)	1 ½ (S)	1 ¾ (S)	1 ¾ (S)
Yogurt, plain	1 ⅓ cup	1 ½ cup	1 ¾ cup	1 ¾ cup	2 cups	2 ¼ cups
Kiwi	½	½	½	⅔	⅔	¾
Peach	½	½	½	⅔	⅔	¾
Apple	½	½	½	⅔	⅔	¾

Directions: Chop kiwi, peach, and apple into bite-size pieces. Mix protein into yogurt. Add fruit.

DAY 13/MEAL 2

Cran-Apple Fun

	1,600	1,800	2,000	2,200	2,400	2,600
Vanilla high alpha whey isolate	1 ½ (S)	2 (S)	2 (S)	2 ½ (S)	2 ⅓ (S)	2 ½ (S)
Cranberries, raw	¾ cup	1 cup	1 cup	1 cup	1 ½ cup	⅓ cup
Apple, medium	1	1	1 ¼	1 ¼	1 ⅓	1 ½
Flaxseed oil	½ tbsp.	⅓ tbsp.	⅓ tbsp.	⅔ tbsp.	½ tbsp.	½ tbsp.
Almonds	½ oz.	½ oz.	⅔ oz.	½ oz.	⅔ oz.	⅔ oz.

Directions: Core apple. In blender, combine cranberries and apple. Blend well. Add protein and flaxseed and blend for additional 10 seconds on low. Eat almonds separately.

DAY 13/MEAL 3

It's a Wrap

	1,600	1,800	2,000	2,200	2,400	2,600
Tortilla, whole-wheat	1	1	1	1	1	1
Chicken breast , skinless	2 oz.	2 oz.	2 ½ oz.	3 oz.	3 oz.	3 oz.
Lettuce, mixed greens	¼ cup	¼ cup	¼ cup	¼ cup	¼ cup	¼ cup
Mozzarella, part-skim	⅛ cup	⅛ cup	⅛ cup	⅛ cup	¼ cup	¼ cup
Mayonnaise	¼ tbsp.	¼ tbsp.	⅓ tbsp.	½ tbsp.	⅓ tbsp.	½ tbsp.
Onion	1 oz.	1 oz.	1 oz.	1 oz.	1 oz.	1 oz.
Tomato	¼	¼	¼	¼	¼	¼
Strawberries	¼ cup	½ cup	½ cup	½ cup	¾ cup	¾ cup
Blueberries	¼ cup	½ cup	½ cup	⅔ cup	¾ cup	1 cup

Directions: Bake chicken breast in oven at 350°F for 30 minutes or until done. Chop chicken, onion, and tomato into bite-size pieces. Grate cheese. Spread mayonnaise over tortilla. Cover with chicken, lettuce, mozzarella, onion, and tomato. Wrap like a fajita. Mix strawberries and blueberries together and eat separately.

DAY 13/MEAL 4

Veggie Protein Surprise

	1,600	1,800	2,000	2,200	2,400	2,600
High alpha whey isolate	1 ½ (S)	2 (S)	2 (S)	2 ½ (S)	2 ⅓ (S)	2 ½ (S)
Vegetable juice (organic)	1 ½ cup	1 ½ cup	1 ½ cup	1 ½ cup	1 ½ cup	1 ½ cup
Flaxseed oil	¾ tbsp.	1 tbsp.	1 tbsp.	1 tbsp.	1 ¼ tbsp.	1 ⅓ tbsp.
Apple	½	½	¾	1	1¼	1 ⅓

Directions: Pour vegetable juice into blender and turn on low speed. Add protein and flaxseed oil and blend for 5-10 seconds. Eat apple separately.

DAY 13/MEAL 5

A Very Veggie Stir-fry

	1,600	1,800	2,000	2,200	2,400	2,600
Tofu	3 ½ oz.	4 oz.	4 oz.	4 ½ oz.	5 oz.	5 oz.
Szechuan sauce	1 ½ tbsp.	2 tbsp.	3 tbsp.	3 tbsp.	3 ½ tbsp.	4 tbsp.
Broccoli	½ cup	½ cup	½ cup	½ cup	½ cup	¾ cup
Carrots	½ cup	½ cup	½ cup	¾ cup	¾ cup	¾ cup
Celery	2	2	2	2	3	3
Bean sprouts	¼ cup	¼ cup	¼ cup	¼ cup	¼ cup	¼ cup
Water chestnuts	¼ cup	¼ cup	¼ cup	¼ cup	¼ cup	¼ cup
Peppers (red or green)	1	1	1	1	1	1
Egg white	1	1	2	2 ½	3	3

Directions: Chop all vegetables into bite-size pieces. Lightly oil skillet. Over medium heat, cook all ingredients except Szechwan sauce and egg . In separate skillet, soft-poach the egg (remove egg yolk prior to poaching). Once vegetables and tofu are cooked, add poached egg, breaking it apart while stirring it in. Add Szechuan sauce.

DAY 14/MEAL 1

The Muse

	1,600	1,800	2,000	2,200	2,400	2,600
Muesli, 5-grain	½ oz.	½ oz.	½ oz.	⅔ oz.	¾ oz.	¾ oz.
Vanilla high alpha whey isolate	1 ½ (S)	1 ½ (S)	1 ½ (S)	1 ½ (S)	2 (S)	2 (S)
Yogurt, plain	½ cup	½ cup	¾ cup	¾ cup	¾ cup	¾ cup
Flaxseed, crushed	½ tsp.	⅔ tsp.	⅔ tsp.	¾ tsp.	¾ tsp.	1 tsp.
Grapefruit	¼	¼	½	½	½	½

Directions: In bowl, combine all ingredients except grapefruit. Eat grapefruit separately.

DAY 14/MEAL 2

Trail Mix

	1,600	1,800	2,000	2,200	2,400	2,600
Chocolate or vanilla high alpha whey isolate	1 ½ (S)	1 ½ (S)	2 (S)	2 (S)	2 ½ (S)	2 ½ (S)
Almonds	⅓ oz.	⅓ oz.	½ oz.	⅔ oz.	⅔ oz.	⅔ oz.
Raisins, seedless	2 oz.	2 oz.	3 oz.	3 oz.	3 ½ oz	3 ½ oz.
Pumpkin seeds	½ oz.	⅔ oz.	½ oz.	⅔ oz.	⅔ oz.	¾ oz.

Directions: In a shaker cup, mix protein with water. Mix almonds, raisins, and pumpkin seeds together.

DAY 14/MEAL 3

Shrimp and Miso

	1,600	1,800	2,000	2,200	2,400	2,600
Rye bread	1	1	1	1	1	1
Cream cheese, light	¼ oz.	⅓ oz.	½ oz.	⅔ oz.	¾ oz.	1 oz.

Cucumber	3 slices	3 slices	3 slices	3 slices	3 slices	3 slices
Tomato	2 slices	2 slices	2 slices	2 slices	2 slices	2 slices
Baby shrimp	¼ cup	⅓ cup	½ cup	½ cup	⅔ cup	⅔ cup
Miso	1 ¾ tbsp.	2 tbsp.	1 ¾ tbsp.	1 ¾ tbsp.	2 tbsp.	3 tbsp.
Tofu, firm	1 ¾ oz.	2 oz.	2 oz.	2oz.	2 oz.	2 oz.
Green onion	½ tbsp.	1 tbsp.	1 tbsp.	1 tbsp.	1 tbsp.	1 tbsp.
Apple	½	½	¾	1	1	1

Directions: In pot, bring 1 ½-3 cups water to a boil. Add miso, tofu, and green onion. Simmer for 20 minutes. Spread cream cheese on toasted rye bread. Top with cucumber, shrimp, and tomato.

DAY 14/MEAL 4

Tahiti Treat

	1,600	1,800	2,000	2,200	2,400	2,600
Frozen yogurt, vanilla	½ cup	½ cup	½ cup	½ cup	½ cup	½ cup
Orange, peeled	¼	¼	½	½	½	½
Pineapple, diced	¼ cup	¼ cup	⅓ cup	⅓ cup	½ cup	½ cup
Banana	¼	¼	⅓	⅓	⅓	½
Water	½ cup	½ cup	½ cup	½ cup	½ cup	½ cup
Vanilla high alpha whey isolate	1½ (S)	2 (S)	2 (S)	2 ½ (S)	2 ½ (S)	2 ½ (S)
Flaxseed oil	½ tsp.	⅔ tsp.	⅔ tsp.	¾ tsp.	1 tsp.	1 tsp.

Directions: In blender, combine orange, pineapple, banana, and frozen yogurt with ½ cup water. Blend well. Add protein and flaxseed, and blend for additional 10 seconds on low.

DAY 14/MEAL 5

Cajun Cod

	1,600	1,800	2,000	2,200	2,400	2,600
Cod	4½ oz.	5 oz.	5 oz.	6 oz.	7 oz.	7 ½ oz.
Olive oil	½ tbsp.	½ tbsp.	⅔ tbsp.	⅔ tbsp.	⅔ tbsp.	¾ tbsp.
Cayenne	¼ tsp.	¼ tsp.	¼ tsp.	¼ tsp.	¼ tsp.	¼ tsp.
Paprika	¼ tsp.	¼ tsp.	¼ tsp.	¼ tsp.	¼ tsp.	¼ tsp.
Oregano	¼ tsp.	¼ tsp.	¼ tsp.	¼ tsp.	¼ tsp.	¼ tsp.
Black pepper	¼ tsp.	¼ tsp.	¼ tsp.	¼ tsp.	¼ tsp.	¼ tsp.
Thyme	¼ tsp.	¼ tsp.	¼ tsp.	¼ tsp.	¼ tsp.	¼ tsp.
Fennel seeds	¼ tsp.	¼ tsp.	¼ tsp.	¼ tsp.	¼ tsp.	¼ tsp.
Mushrooms, Shiitake	¾ cup	¾ cup	¾ cup	¾ cup	1 cup	1 cup
Garlic clove	1	1	1	1	1	1
Butter	⅓ tbsp.	½ tbsp.	½ tbsp.	⅔ tbsp.	⅔ tbsp.	¾ tbsp.
Red wine	3 oz.	3 oz.	4 oz.	4 oz.	4 oz.	4 ½ oz.

Directions: *Cod*: Combine all spices in a bowl. Using your hands, cover one side of the fillets with spices. In skillet, warm oil on medium-high heat and cook cod, spice side down, for approximately 2 minutes (until browned). Turn cod over and bake in the oven at 400°F for additional 5 minutes. Fish will be flaky when done. *Mushrooms*: Slice mushrooms. In skillet over medium heat, melt butter. Crush garlic and add to butter. Add mushrooms and cook until done. Enjoy wine with meal.

Recommended Food Swaps for Vegetarians: Even though the recommended meal plans are not necessarily vegetarian-based, there are many ways in which vegetarians can easily and healthfully incorporate their favorite protein foods. Many of the meals will suit an active lacto-ovo-vegetarian (those who consume milk and eggs but no meat) lifestyle. Not all macronutrient quantities will match those of meat-based products. Please use discretion when planning your Fat Wars meals around these foods.

VEGETARIAN SWAPS				
	Calories	**Protein**	**Fat**	**Carbs**
Soy-protein isolate: 1 serving	100	25 g	0 g	0 g
Tofu (extra firm): 3 oz.	55	7 g	2 g	2 g
Tempeh: ½ cup	165	16 g	6 g	14 g
Veggie ground round: ⅓ cup	85	11 g	2.5 g	4.6 g
Veggie dogs: 1	46	9 g	0 g	1 g
Hot and Spicy Chili Veggie Dogs: 1	74	13 g	1.1 g	2.7 g
Jumbo Veggie Dogs: 1	104	16 g	1.3 g	6.8 g
Garden Vegetable Patties: 1	80	9.5 g	0.9 g	10 g
The Good Veggie Burger: 1	105	12 g	4 g	6.9 g
Veggie Bologna Slices: 62 g	81	15 g	0.9 g	3.5 g
Veggie Salami Slices: 62 g	66	17 g	0.4 g	4.5 g
Veggie Turkey Slices: 62 g	85	15 g	1.7 g	4.4 g
Veggie Ham Slices: 62 g	80	1g	0.2 g	6 g
(Yves Veggie Cuisine products)				

Fat Wars on the Town

Looking for the keys to eating out and being sociable without blowing your Fat Wars eating strategy completely? Your success at fighting the war on fat is largely determined by your lifestyle and dietary choices. In fact, every time you sit down to eat you are either moving one step closer to winning your Fat War—or one step closer to losing it. Each day, and perhaps each hour, you are empowered to make a choice that advances your goals or sets them back.

Too often I hear people talking about the things they should not do in order to improve their lives. But the real magic lies in approaching our daily goals with a positive attitude. In other words, it is better to focus on things we will do to improve our lives rather than things we shouldn't do. The difference is subtle, yet the outcome can be quite profound.

Since it has taken most of us many years to transform into the shape and health we are presently experiencing, we cannot expect positive transformation overnight. One fat-promoting meal easily turns into a second and so on, just as one day of lethargy turns into a second and so on. We all have choices. Unfortunately, too many of us take the easy road and end up breaking down long before we reach the end.

It is not always easy to make the right choices in life, but the bottom line is we all have to live with whatever choices we make. Some of the hardest choices come in the form of what and when to eat when we are on the road. Quite frequently, we may be making food choices unconsciously in an effort to satisfy a need that is not tangible at the time. We need to be preemptive and make sure we plan for behaviors and situations, so we are always one step ahead in the Fat Wars.

Part of a winning strategy is anticipating the situations that will trigger old behaviors of eating. To help you avoid defeating behaviors, I will provide you with scenarios that suggest how to stay on the Fat Wars program when eating out, during different social situations, and on the road.

Being on the Fat Wars program is about making changes that will transform your life. It is not a plan designed to keep you from enjoying social situations; it is a plan that allows you to enjoy the fruits of life with proper food choices that allow you to live a healthier lifestyle while becoming leaner in the process. It will make you rethink some of the behaviors that did not fare well for you in the past and will help you continue to build on the positive behaviors you already engage in.

Restaurants

In spite of our good intentions to make healthful meals, our lives are filled with competing interests that draw us to making convenient choices. When eating out either at a stylish restaurant or fast-food outlet, consider these strategies:

- When you have a choice, choose a restaurant that provides you with a varied menu. Stay away from menus that do not allow you to make a healthful choice. Some examples include fish-and-chip restaurants, fried-chicken outlets, and barbecued-rib restaurants.

- While at the restaurant, be strategic and choose foods that are wholesome instead of processed. These unprocessed foods will not only provide you with the greatest amount of nutrients but also keep you full with the least number of calories.

- Ask yourself questions when you are making a food choice at a restaurant. How much unhealthy fat does the food have? Does it contain good fats or bad ones? Fats provide the most calories for the lowest amount of nutrients. This is an important area to consider when you decide how much and what type of fat you will consume. By making the right choice you may be cutting your total number of calories in half.

- When you sit down at a restaurant, a basket of bread gets brought to the table. Start by asking the waiter not to serve the bread at your table, as it is best to avoid the temptation altogether. There are practically no restaurants that serve healthful, stone-ground or sprouted-grain breads, so it is best to just say no. Eating the bread will stimulate a fat-storing high-insulin response, add calories to your meal, yet provide you with very little nutrient density. If you are in a situation where others at your table want bread, do your very best to avoid eating any of it.

- Make sure you choose a main dish that is not starch-based. Choose meals that are high in protein and low in starchy carbohydrates. Most restaurants are very accommodating, so don't be afraid to ask the waiter for the type of meal that is most conducive to fat burning. In other words, you do not always have to have exactly what the menu lists.

- Make sure to include a good portion of fibrous mixed vegetables with your protein source. For instance, if you are ordering steak, chicken, or fish, try to forgo the baked potato or rice pilaf for a nice serving of veggies.

Here are some simple suggestions that will help you eat a healthier Fat Wars friendly meal at a restaurant:

- Ask for dressings and sauces on the side rather than on top of the foods you order.

- Opt for broth, fruit, or vegetable-based sauces rather than creamy sauces.

- Always say no to the tempting bread.

- Choose meals that are poached, steamed, broiled, or baked, but never fried.

- Choose fruits or yogurt-based desserts. Have the occasional dark chocolate treat, but make that treat infrequent and small.

Foods that contain more fibers tend to fill you up and control the release of your fat-storing hormone, insulin. Therefore:

- Avoid refined rice and any white-flour products, including pasta.

- Go for large amounts and a wide variety of vegetables. If necessary ask for a larger portion of your favorite vegetable.

- Remember to ask for steamed, broiled, baked, or poached vegetables that are not lathered in butter but lightly coated with olive oil. There are fewer calories in vegetables because they contain large amounts of water.

Don't be deceived by the belief that beverages don't contain calories just because they don't contain fat. Alcohol can contain an enormous number calories and make you feel hungry rather than provide you with valuable nutrients. Here are a few valuable rules to follow:

- Always have water as your beverage of choice at a restaurant.

- Mix some fresh lemon or lime into your water for taste and health-promoting alkalinity.

- And go for the glass of red wine once in a while. After all, you are human, aren't you?

Even while traveling:

- Don't use different life scenarios as an excuse not to follow the Fat Wars plan. Even when you are on the road, make sure you are always prepared by having a healthful snack on hand. Bring or buy fresh vegetables and fruit, protein powder, and water.

- At the airport, stay away from fast-food restaurants. I have yet to find an airport restaurant that complies with any of the Fat Wars strategies.

- Always bring plenty of water with you on the plane. It will keep you satisfied, and refresh you and prevent you from dehydrating.

- Being on the road can be an exciting as well as a challenging time. Many events may trigger your old eating behaviors. Avoid situations where you might to eat in a way that will not enable you to achieve your goals.

- When at a hotel, ask for a room with a fridge, or book into a hotel that contains a kitchenette. Purchase as much of your own food as possible to ensure adherence to the Fat Wars strategies.

A Few More Points

I spoke earlier about the importance of setting up an environment conducive to achieving your goals. Start when you are grocery shopping. Examine the labels of foods that are unfamiliar to you, and avoid foods that are highly refined and contain a lot of sodium and hydrogenated fat. Remember that ingredients are listed by amount most predominant. Choose foods that contain natural ingredients and ingredients you recognize. By stocking your cupboards, fridge, and freezer with appropriate food choices, you will ensure success.

Part of setting up an optimal environment is surrounding yourself with people who will help you achieve your goal of fat loss. Talk honestly with family and friends and let them know how they can be supportive and champion your success. Encourage them to join you in your quest for a healthier life.

When invited to social situations, offer to bring a dish that you can enjoy at the party. Prepare a healthy dish so you have an alternative. Eat before you attend the function so you will not find yourself hungry and vulnerable. During the celebration choose foods such as raw vegetables, salads, and fruit- and vegetable-based dishes. Avoid fried foods at any cost.

When you go to the movies, don't go hungry. If at all possible have a couple of cups of air-popped popcorn before you go. Take some breath mints with you to help you stay away from movie theater popcorn, and drink lots of water to keep your mind off food.

Last and most important, remember that you are human, and there will be a time or two that you may stray away from your plan. Remember to forgive yourself, and remember you have the power to get back on the plan with your very next meal. That is the real beauty behind hormonal eating with Fat Wars. You are only as good—hormonally speaking—as the last meal you consumed. Try to ensure a proper fat-burning environment as often as possible.

TRANSFORMING THROUGH BIOCIZE

Introduction

For many people, exercise can seem like one of the most complicated subjects. There are gyms—with their bulky equipment and inflated, fast-talking staff members. And, please let's not forget the infomercials! Sets, repetitions, frequency of exercise sessions, duration, speed of movement, time between sets—it can be intimidating enough to leave you scratching your head as the only form of exercise you end up doing. No wonder so many people quit before they ever see results. Everyone seems to have the answers. When to exercise, what to do, where to do it, and how long to do it for. If that's not enough, there's all that high-tech state-of-the-art machinery to contend with. Is it really worth the effort? And why does everyone seem to know what they're doing? Everyone except for you!

Introducing Biocize, A New Concept in Training Progress

The by-product of proper exercise really is worth the effort you put in, especially where the Fat Wars are concerned. But the important thing to remember is *proper exercise*, which in the Fat Wars program is referred to as Biocize. It's a training concept that was born out of the realization that many of the changes in body composition and health status that have been deemed the normal result of aging (for example, loss of muscle and gain in body fat) are instead the result of a long-standing sedentary lifestyle or improper exercise.

The concepts surrounding Biocize were developed after researching the most effective exercise strategies (including timing, duration, hormonal elevations, and nutrient partitioning) for positively affecting one's biological status from a hormonal perspective. As you are now aware, hormones are our key cellular messengers, and losing key messages through the decline of certain fundamental hormones is one of the causes of the body transformation many have come to fear past middle age. That negative transformation is also directly responsible for robbing us of our youth and prematurely aging us.

The two most important hormones when it comes to the body's ability to increase its lean body mass and burn its excess fat stores are human growth hormone (HGH) and testosterone (yes, even for you ladies). Both HGH and testosterone decline precipitously through the aging cycle, and as we witness their decline we also witness the increase of many of the disorders associated with lost muscle mass, including excess body fat, loss of strength, and loss of energy and vitality. Without the message of repair and renewal—called anabolism—obtained through the synergy of these two hormones, we most certainly can expect to succumb to the Smaller Fat Person syndrome.

The goal of Biocize is to first enhance the stimulation of these hormones through the right type of exercise. The program is based on revolutionary and scientifically sound concepts that are designed to increase the functionality of your body. The truth—which most people forget—is that the structure of our bodies is extremely complicated, but its function is not. As humans, we are constantly engaged in four common forces: we push, pull, lift, and carry. It stands to reason that our exercise training should involve the very forces we utilize day in and day out (pushing, pulling, lifting, and carrying).

This exercise program is designed to allow you to gain maximal muscle while maintaining an effective fat-burning metabolism. The exercises laid out in this chapter are created around the four forces mentioned above. One example of everyday use of these four forces can be found in something you probably never give a thought to, the motion of walking. While walking, you push off one foot, lift that leg up, pull it forward to strike the ground again, and carry it through to repeat the walking phase.

Unfortunately, when it comes to resistance training—training with weights—especially in a gym or fitness center, the industry has traditionally dictated what occurs in the exercise setting. Sometimes it seems those dysfunctional machines were designed for everyone but us. They are either too small or too big, the motion is not always fluid, and we never seem to feel the muscles the machine tells us we should feel. And more often then not, the machinery seems to be scattered all over the gym. Biocize is designed differently. The Biocize exercise programs are custom-designed for the human body, not a machine.

Equipment

The exercises incorporate functional resistance training movements using your own body weight, dumbbells, barbells, or anything you can find around your house that has enough resistance. (Soup cans may even serve as a starting point!) You will gain not only the strength and lean body mass associated with resistance training, but also the ability to control your body and improve your movement. You will see consistent improvements in your body. This allows you to move ever forward. You won't hit sticking points.

When you strap yourself into a conventional exercise machine and start pumping away, you *isolate* certain muscles. In the bodybuilding world, bigger muscles tend to have a positive connotation. But Biocize involves integrating movements for maximum hormonal strength, muscular strength, and metabolic enhancement. In your everyday activities, you integrate muscular contractions to create movements in a controlled and balanced fashion. On a strength machine, you do not challenge your balance or coordination, and each muscle is trained in isolation. Why not get more bang for your buck by integrating movements? You will develop more muscle in less time, your metabolic cost will be higher, and there will be a greater hormonal benefit because you are affecting more tissues! What does all this mean to you? A better body with greater fat-burning engines, that's what!

Everyone has a different starting point in the Biocize exercise journey. Some people have been involved with physical activity all their lives, while for many, being yelled at in eighth-grade gym class was enough abuse. In Biocize, your past exercise experience (both good and bad) is referred to as your training age.

The exercises are selected with this in mind. You can select a resistance and intensity that is unique to you. There are also several progressions. You can progress from your first six-week transformation to another, and another, keeping in mind that you *have completed* or *will be completing* the Fat Wars 45 Day Transformation Program.

The Aerobics Myth

One of the first things people think of when trying to lose excess weight is performing endless hours of aerobic exercise. It's no wonder people get so discouraged when trying to lose excess body fat. *Aerobic* refers to the use of oxygen. The person performing aerobic exercises—jogging, step aerobics, or skipping rope—is forcing the body to use more oxygen. By using extra oxygen, the body draws upon its fat reserves for a great deal of the workout energy. People still believe aerobics is the optimum form of fat-burning exercise. Aerobic activity definitely has its place in a health-enhancing program, but the fact remains that for every person who has won the war against fat using only aerobics, there are fifty others who have not. Permanent fat loss is a fleeting dream for those who use only aerobic means to obtain it.

For many people, aerobic workouts are too long, and the fat burned during the workout is minimal. As in dieting and fasting, the engines that burn the fat—muscle tissue—are burned up, too, and the increase in the amount of fat burned before the next workout is almost zip. Research confirms that excess aerobics causes overtraining and muscle wasting, and anything that strips the body of its metabolically active tissue becomes a rate-limiting step in fat loss.

Build Muscle, Burn Fat

Unlike aerobics, resistance training creates the need for the body to rebuild and repair itself in a process referred to as anabolism.

Anabolism means enhanced muscle mass and function, and you should know by now that your muscle tissue can either make you or break you in the Fat Wars. Biocize is not about building muscle size. Instead it is about enhancing muscle function so that your muscle cells become fat-burning machines. I know it sounds funny, but the muscles you presently have can be tuned up to become more efficient at burning fat. The right type of exercise—Biocize—can do that for you.

The activity of your muscle cells dictates the rate at which your metabolic engines run. If you are carrying around too much extra fat, your muscle tissue has been somewhat deactivated, and it needs a tune-up. The more muscle you rebuild, repair, and train to function at a higher capacity, the more fat you burn within a twenty-four-hour period. One pound of active muscle can burn almost 50 calories a day. So, if you add muscle during your fat-loss program—or at least keep the muscle you have and train it to become more metabolically active—you will be well on your way to winning the Fat Wars.

Biocize is all about balance between resistance training and cardio exercise. Many studies prove the theory that resistance training synergized with low-impact cardio is superior to either one alone. One study, presented in the prestigious *American Journal of Cardiology*, compared aerobic training to aerobic-with-resistance (weight) training. Participants were split into two groups and had to complete a ten-week exercise program. One group completed 75 minutes of aerobic exercise twice a week, while the other completed 40 minutes of aerobics, plus 35 minutes of weight training. At the end of the study, the aerobics group had an 11% increase in endurance, but no increase in their strength. The group that completed the combination of aerobics and resistance training showed a 109% increase in their endurance and a 21% to 43% increase in their overall strength. Both groups spent the same amount of time exercising. The types of exercise they performed played a great role in their success.

Too many people make the mistake of increasing their cardio activity when they don't see the fat melting off their bodies from the usual aerobic load. But the more cardio you do in the absence of proper resistance exercise, the less fat you seem to burn, due to the law of diminished returns. One problem is that excess cardio activity can eat away at muscle tissue. And the more cardio you do, the fewer calories become used in the activity. How can this be, you ask. Doesn't it make sense that the more activity you perform the more calories you burn? Only to a certain degree.

Your body has the ability—over time—to perform the same amount of exercise but burn fewer calories in the process. This is a process of adaptation we have inherited, right along with our 30 billion fat cells. By continuously performing aerobic exercise in the absence of proper resistance, you end up munching on your own muscle tissue, especially around the 90-minutes-of-continuous-cardio mark. And your body will shut down its fat-burning systems, as well. The body does this by slowing the release of fat-mobilizing enzymes and hormones, instead opting for sugar and protein from muscle tissue. So in a very real sense, those people who feel they need to work harder and harder to burn the fat are *adding* to their fat reserves in the end. Talk about a waste of energy.

How Hard Do We Have to Work to Burn Fat?

Fats are made up of many single units called fatty acids. Each individual fatty acid must first be broken apart in order to contribute its energy value. Just as a log burns best in a high-oxygen atmosphere, so do your fatty acids. The problem is that people equate more oxygen to gasping for air during exercise. Nothing could be further from the truth. Forget about your target heart rate, and forget about stopping to take your pulse. Forget the mathematical equations people tell you to solve so you can burn fat while performing aerobic exercise. Here's a simple formula to remember.

The minute you start to gasp for air while exercising, your body switches gears and starts burning sugar and amino acids from muscle tissue as its main fuel. If you can't carry on a conversation while exercising, then you're burning sugar and protein instead of fat. Gasping is an indication that insufficient oxygen is being supplied to the tissues. It takes an enormous amount of fuel to burn the dense fat molecules. When there isn't enough oxygen, your body switches to fuels other than fat. Remember, body fat is very dense, and it requires a great deal of oxygen to be burned as fuel. The optimal intensity when it comes to fat loss is *whatever intensity allows you to take in enough oxygen to burn fat*, which is excellent news for all of you who love taking long walks— an excellent fat-burning exercise.

How Long Is Too Long in Biocize?

The majority of exercisers these days are much too concerned about the number of calories being burned during their exercise activities. By concentrating our efforts on this aspect of training, it's easy to exercise too long. So in a very real sense, we can do too much exercise just as easily as we can do too little.

Time spent away from the gym can be more beneficial to your fat-burning efforts than time spent in it. Cardio and weight-bearing activity won't burn a great deal of fat during the exercise sessions. The real magic lies in their ability to raise your resting metabolic rate—the rate at which you burn calories at rest—for most of the day. One study showed that more than two-thirds of the fat-burning activity of exercise takes place after the actual exercise sessions. This increase in fat-burning potential has been shown to last more than 15 hours in highly trained athletes. Approximately 15 minutes after completing Biocize, your anabolic hormones, testosterone, and growth hormone begin to rise. As long as you don't blunt this anabolic increase by consuming the wrong foods, your body will have the ability to burn extra fat for many hours to come.

The Optimum Duration of Cardio in Biocize

You already know that gasping for air is a no-no when you perform the aerobic portion of Biocize. Do you know the length of time needed to effectively burn fat? The answer is less than 90 minutes of lower impact, and no more than 20 to 30 minutes of high intensity, once your fitness profile changes for the better.

Your body is like an engine on a cold day when you begin to exercise—it needs time to warm up. Fat is not the starting fuel for cold bodies. The body usually starts warming up with a rich sugar mix instead. In order to change the primary fuel to fat, the body must first call into action hormonal and enzymatic responses. Remember: hormones are those tiny, scurrying chemical messengers that give orders to the cells; enzymes are responsible for carrying out the orders.

Once these hormonal and enzymatic troopers are fully on the scene, the fatty acids can be delivered—by special carrier proteins—to the muscle cells and escorted into the furnaces of those cells to be burned as energy. This biochemical fat-burning response (depending on a host of variables such as undigested food and nutrients) usually takes women at least 20 minutes to accomplish. Men need a little less time.

Keeping the Engine Revved

There are two things we can do to compensate for the 20-minute start-up for effective fat loss. 1) Do the cardio activity longer than 20 minutes to increase the fat-burning effect. 2) Do the cardio activity after the resistance portion. Doing cardio right after weight training is like getting into a warmed-up vehicle. All you have to do is turn up the heat, and voilà! A blast of warm air. This warm air is a metaphor for the way your body reacts to aerobic activity after resistance activity. Your fatty acids are readily available as a fuel source—right from the start. This is especially true if your muscles have been used regularly over a certain period of time. It takes, on average, about fifteen days to convert your metabolism from a sugar-burning one to a fat-burning one. Conditioned muscles are very effective at using fat as an energy source.

The Optimum Duration of Resistance Exercise

We need to create some physical stress to increase the levels of free fatty acids in the bloodstream, but too much can cause a drastic increase in cortisol—the muscle-wasting hormone. When it comes to proper resistance training, less can often mean more in terms of progress. Soon after *forty-five minutes* of continuous weight-bearing exercise, levels of cortisol (the major stress hormone) rise so much that recovery from the exercise can become blunted. Excess cortisol is responsible for stealing valuable nitrogen from muscle tissue and turning the amino acids into sugar to create extra energy. The more cortisol produced, the harder it is to get rid of, and the worse off you are for it.

CALORIES BURNED HAVING FUN

This chart gives you an idea of how many calories a 150-pound person would burn in 1 hour of each activity. You can see from the chart that you're probably not burning as many calories in the gym as you might hope. When you do something you enjoy, you're often not thinking about the calories being expended, but instead about the fun you're having. Ultimately, doing something fun is the best way to burn calories on a regular basis.

ACTIVITY	CALORIES BURNED
Aerobic exercise, moderate intensity	350
Bicycling or stationary cycling (10 mph)	415
Hiking with a 20-lb backpack (3 mph)	400
Roller-skating	350
Dancing	350
Treadmill walking (4 mph)	345
Calisthenics	300
Rowing machine, low intensity	300
Rowing machine, moderate intensity	655
Golf, walking with clubs	270
Walking, mild (2 to 2.5 mph)	185 to 255
Walking, vigorous (5 mph)	555
Stair-climbing machine	680
Rope jumping	660
Step aerobics, moderate intensity	610
Cross-country skiing (5 mph)	600
Swimming	540

The Best Time to Exercise

Now that you are acquainted with the importance, intensity, duration, and sequence of Biocize, you need to learn the optimum time to perform it for the greatest fat-burning value. Many people exercise too late in the day. I don't know how they do it. This is the time we walk into our local gym and have to take a number just to use the equipment. Exercising in the evening after a hard workday can be detrimental for a number of reasons. After a day of work we have little energy left for a workout. It's hard enough making dinner after work, let alone exercising. Our motivation at this time is usually low, due to lowered dopamine and serotonin levels, and many people will come up with myriad excuses to avoid exercising. The problem is, it gets easier and easier to miss a workout, and before we know it we're right back at the starting block again.

Exercising in the evening also increases those pesky fat-stripping stress hormones. This is the time when they should be at their lowest. These stress hormones not only can keep us awake—they also interfere with our recuperation, ultimately slowing down fat loss.

The best time to exercise for the greatest fat-burning buck is first thing in the morning. "First thing in the morning, are you crazy?" I know: you barely have enough energy to get out of bed in the morning. If you were to lie down on an exercise bench you'd probably fall asleep. Trust me, once your body gets used to the new schedule, you'll never want to train at any other time.

When you adapt yourself to earlier training, you allow yourself to take advantage of your body's higher metabolic rate—for the entire day. Every time you sit down to eat after exercising, your body will be more efficient at burning the calories from the food you consume all day long. Unless you have no choice, why would you want to lose this advantage by exercising in the evening?

Should I Eat Before I Exercise?

Any way you look at it, exercising—even Biocize—is stressful on the body, which is why the body responds by elevating certain stress hormones such as adrenaline and cortisol. When the body is stressed, its last priority is digesting food. The majority of the blood supply is ushered to the extremities, away from the stomach.

This is why I do not recommend consuming a great deal of solid food before exercise; most of it will just sit there fermenting in your gut. Instead, try training yourself to exercise on an empty stomach, or with a limited amount of food (between 100 to 150 calories) consumed about 30 to 45 minutes before Biocize.

The worst food to consume before exercising is a high-glycemic carbohydrate source such as dry cereal. The quick-breakdown carbs will raise your insulin levels and cause you to use glucose (sugar) as your primary fuel instead of fat. The best food to consume before exercising is a liquid protein shake with an easily digestible whey isolate, soy isolate, or a mix of the two. High-protein liquid meals empty from the stomach quickly, causing a rise in the hormone glucagon (the primary hormone for maintaining glucose levels during exercise), allowing for enhanced fat-burning activity. So if you must eat something before exercise, make it a protein shake with water, and keep it to around 100 calories (see Appendix for recommendations).

What About After Biocize?

After exercise, especially the weight-training portion, the body requires refueling of its glycogen (short-term energy) reserves. To make sure this happens, the body contains an enzyme called glycogen synthetase, which is responsible for storing sugar for future needs. Within a 2-hour window after exercise, this enzyme is extra hungry. This 2-hour window is the only time you can consume larger-than-normal amounts of higher-glycemic carbohydrates without worrying that they'll convert to fat.

Many of us make the mistake of consuming only carbohydrates, for example, fruit juice, after a workout. Drinking carbohydrate beverages without consuming sufficient protein after exercising causes a drastic increase in insulin levels. The insulin depresses growth hormone and testosterone levels. Research confirms that protein mixed with carbohydrates after training allows for faster muscle recovery and greater increases in growth hormone and testosterone.

For best results, as soon after completing your workout as possible, mix protein with carbohydrates in a liquid form to insure rapid replacement of bodily sugars and protein for recovery. See Section II for recipes.

Biocize Muscle–Building, Fat–Burning Exercise Rules

There are right and wrong ways to perform Biocize. If you follow the tips presented in this section, I guarantee that your progress will be greatly enhanced. These principles have been gathered from my extensive background in the fitness-sciences field:

- **Always warm up**. A cold muscle is an unactivated muscle. It won't give you much performance, and it can be damaged if you push it too hard. Always take 10 to 15 minutes to warm up the body. Walking on a treadmill or peddling on a stationary bike are two good activities that will get the blood pumping. I do not recommend stretching right off the bat, since stretching a cold muscle can cause injury to that muscle. If you want to stretch, warm the muscle group first and then stretch.

- **Technique is everything**, **especially when you're weight lifting**. If I had a dollar for every time I saw someone training improperly, I'd be a lot better off than I am today. People seem to be in such a hurry when they work out, lifting weights improperly. Most of the time, these people don't pay attention to the exercise they are performing. If you want to see results fast, then pay close attention to the way you perform your exercises. Follow the Biocize guidelines as closely as possible—your success on the program depends greatly on the tempo of the exercises.

- **Always cool down after completion**. This is the opportune time to stretch. Take about 10 minutes at the end of the routine to cool down properly. When stretching, make sure you move into the stretch slowly, breathing deeply the entire time. Hold the stretch for at least 10 seconds, and preferably 30 seconds to 1 minute. Then slowly come back to the starting position. Most people stretch improperly, which does nothing for the muscle except damage it. Stretching will also help to remove excess lactic acid produced during the weight-training phase of Biocize.

Different Muscle Fibers for Different Functions

Below you will find information on two different kinds of muscle fibers that form your musculature. We all have both types, but we all have them in different ratios. The difference in performance ability of athletes can be measured in the amount of each type of muscle fiber that dominates their physiology:

- **Type I** slow-twitch muscle fibers use oxygen to produce a steady supply of energy. The fibers function more slowly than their fast-twitch counterparts and are best suited for non-intensive aerobic activities because they do not tire easily. These muscle fibers have large numbers of capillaries (small blood vessels) that are used to transport oxygen and nutrients into the muscle cells and remove waste products like carbon dioxide. Athletes who excel at endurance activities have a higher percentage of these fibers.

- **Type II** fast-twitch muscles do not have as high a need for oxygen, so they function well in an anaerobic (low-oxygen) environment. These muscle fibers can contract rapidly and do very well in high-intensity situations where strength and speed are needed. They are ideally suited for low-endurance activities that require quick bursts of energy, such as weight lifting, sprinting, or jumping. They are also called into use during many stop-and-go sports, such as basketball and volleyball. The fast-twitch muscle fibers tire quickly because of the increase in lactic acid, a by-product of anaerobic environments. Athletes who excel at short-duration, high-intensity activities seem to have a larger percentage of fast-twitch muscles.

On the Go

To maintain great results on the program, you must perform Biocize regularly. If you travel, plan on exercising while on the road. If you can't get a hotel with a gym, you can still find alternate ways to do many of the exercises. Whether you use elastic bands, soup cans, or special vinyl dumbbells that can be filled with water, you will be able to complete a decent enough workout to maintain results. Remember, everything counts! A little workout is better than no workout.

If you feel intimidated and self-conscious training at a health club, remember that others training alongside you will respect you for being there. They know that what you're trying to accomplish is something millions of couch potatoes are avoiding. No one will make fun of you or condemn you for fighting the good fight. Look around, and you will notice many—if not most—people there look just like you.

If you can't afford a gym membership, or you're too intimidated to train with others, or it takes too much of your time, or you just like to train by yourself, then consider training at home or outdoors. You don't have to use the fancy equipment found in a gym for great results on Biocize, although I think it helps. You can buy an inexpensive barbell set or a set of adjustable dumbbells from your local mass retailer or sporting-goods store for under $60. You can also use other items around your house, such as a couple of old cans (from soup to paint, as you get more fit) filled with water or sand.

Be Active All Day Long

Even though Biocize is a very efficient means to get and stay in shape, you also need to train yourself to be more active every chance you get. Every single little thing you may take for granted counts. Every time you take the stairs instead of the elevator, every time you choose a parking space a little farther from the mall, and every time you play with your kids instead of saying "I'm too tired" counts!

Important Points to Remember

- Don't expect to see the new you overnight. We seem to forget the road that got us here in the first place. We didn't wake up one morning to suddenly discover layers of fat on our formerly buff physiques. We got here one Twinkie and one sedentary day at a time.

- Give yourself sufficient time to reach your goals, an ounce of fat at a time.

- What you did in the past doesn't count. You may be skeptical that this new exercise plan is going to work when everything else failed. If applied correctly, Biocize will provide quite the boost to your fat-burning arsenal.

- You must become self-motivated to succeed. The best way to get into the habit of regular exercise is through plenty of practice, beginning with the exercises outlined in *Fat Wars: 45 Days to Transform Your Body*.

- You must change your attitude toward exercise. People who view an exercise routine as a chore instead of a meaningful part of their life will not succeed for very long. There will always be times you won't be able to exercise. But more often than not, something that prohibits you from training is in your mind. Don't put off exercise for one more minute—your transformation depends on it.

- Apply the strategies you learn here as if they were the last detail to your fat-loss battle plan, because they are. Without exercising, you will fall short of your objectives. And even if you lose weight, you will likely gain it all back, and then some. Is that what you really want? Or would you rather lose the fat and keep it off permanently? I thought so.

Program Variables

1. Sets and Repetitions

"Sets" refers to the number of groups of exercises you will perform in one exercise session. "Repetitions" refers to the number of single efforts you attempt to do in succession. For example, if the program calls for two sets of eight repetitions, you would perform eight repetitions of the movement before stopping. You would then attempt another eight repetitions.

The number of sets and repetitions you perform ultimately determines your *volume*. For example, a program prescribing three sets of ten repetitions will give you thirty repetitions in total for the exercise. You will have performed thirty repetitions, with a resistance that was manageable for ten repetitions at a time.

You could achieve the same volume by doing six sets of five repetitions. You would perform thirty repetitions with a resistance that was manageable for five repetitions at a time. Let's compare the two examples: you would be exercising at a higher intensity for the same amount of total volume of repetitions.

It is common in the exercise world to hear people complaining about their exercise programs. The main complaint is the inability to see consistent results from a program. This often happens if we perform the same exercises in the same manner over and over again. In Biocize, the repetitions vary to change the stimulus and continue to force the body to adapt. Remember, when exercising, your body is doing its best to adapt, and once it does, your old workout will no longer challenge you to make changes! We have to adjust the sets, resistance, rest, and, of course, the repetitions. In fact, strength expert Charles Poliquin of Montreal, coach to many top NHL and NFL athletes, feels that the number of repetitions is the variable to which the exerciser adapts most quickly.

Biocize is all about transformation. To help you see and feel a total transformation, Biocize considers the effect certain hormones play in relation to specific forms of exercise. Hormones are the key cellular messengers. Losing key messages through the decline of certain fundamental hormones as we age is one of the biological markers of aging itself. By increasing the hormones that decline through the aging cycle, we may be able to mimic the message of youth.

Two of the top biomarkers (physiological markers) of aging are the loss of lean body mass (muscle, bone, tissue) and the loss of strength. In a groundbreaking study presented in the *Journal of the American Medical Association* in 1990, muscle size and strength were greatly improved in as little as eight weeks of resistance training, even in ninety-year-old subjects. If a ninety-year-old can do it, what do you think you are capable of? There is no doubt that proper resistance training, which maximizes the benefits of the hormones testosterone, human growth hormone (HGH), and IGF-1, is the most effective kind of exercise for building muscle, increasing strength, and melting body fat.

Much research points to the fact that through increased levels of these three hormones, we can expect to see the greatest transformation. One such study, carried out in 1997 by Dr. L. A. Gotshalk and colleagues, was published in the *Canadian Journal of Applied Physiology*. The study demonstrated that multiple sets of exercises were more effective in elevating testosterone, growth hormone, and IGF-1 than a single set of each exercise. In this study, exercisers were involved in either single-set heavy-resistance exercise or three sets of heavy-resistance exercise. When the relative increases of the aforementioned hormones were assessed for each protocol (single or multiple), the three-set protocol produced significant elevations immediately following the exercises and increased steadily for up to 60 minutes thereafter. When we compare this to the single-set protocol, where elevations were only seen immediately and up to 15 minutes afterward, we see our motivation to perform those extra sets! In Biocize, your exercise program will vary from performing two sets to as many as four, but don't be worried. You'll be done before your body knows what hit it!

2. Tempo

The speed of movement during an exercise is referred to as the tempo. Unfortunately, tempo is often overlooked in an exercise program. Poor tempo is one of the main reasons exercisers do not experience continued results. When it comes to overall success on an exercise plan, tempo is one of the most important variables to consider. Tempo determines the *time under tension*, which highly influences the body's response to the exercise. When you intentionally slow the pace of an exercise repetition, you place more emphasis on proper form and leave less room for error or injury.

For example, if you were to perform two sets of eight repetitions of an exercise at a fast pace, each set might take 20 seconds. By contrast, if the movements were performed at a more controlled pace, a set would likely take 40 to 60 seconds or more to perform. This will make a significant difference in how your training will affect you. (See Tempo Determines the Set's Duration for more detail.)

Biocize illustrates the tempo for each exercise by indicating (in seconds) the speed of movement for each movement in the exercise. For example, if you were to perform a pressing movement away from the body, the program may indicate "2 up/4 down." This means that when you press against gravity, you should take 2 seconds to complete the movement, pause at the midpoint for 1 second, and take 4 seconds to return the weight with gravity. This would be one repetition. Before completing the next repetition, you would pause at the start point, then begin again, taking 2 seconds to press against gravity.

Here's an example:
Dumbbell Chest Press   2 sets   8 repetitions   2 up/4 down

In this example, the exerciser will press the dumbbells off the chest (against gravity) for approximately 2 seconds, counting "one, two." Once the arms are extended, the exerciser will hold the dumbbells for 1 second before lowering the weight (with gravity), counting "one, two, three, four." Before beginning the next repetition, the exerciser will pause for 1 second. Each repetition takes 7 seconds to complete, and the whole set will take about 60 seconds to finish.

Tempo Determines the Set's Duration (Time under Tension)

Tempo will have a great effect on how long it takes to perform each set. I'll explain why this concept is important and why each exercise is performed for 40 to 60 seconds.

Sets that last approximately 40 to 60 seconds will use more energy to replenish the substrates (energy substances) within the muscle cells. This *energy cost* increases the amount of calories you burn. Why? Because more work is being performed!

Very short sets of exercises, say 20 seconds, use readily available energy stores to get the job completed. With longer sets, the body starts out the same way, using readily available energy stores, but then progresses by providing the necessary energy—such as glucose and amino acids—for muscle contractions.

These longer sets will also produce hormone-elevating by-products such as lactic acid. This substance is produced when a muscle contraction lasts longer than 20 to 30 seconds. Then the lactic acid is broken down and removed in another *energy-costing* process; this time glucose and fatty acids fuel the process.

Times of approximately 20 to 30 seconds per set will cause few changes in lean body mass, but will cause changes in absolute strength. But times of 40 to 60 seconds per set will influence positive *hypertrophy* (increases in lean muscle mass) of both types of muscle fibers. This way, we are able to train for an increase in lean muscle mass of all types of muscle fibers. This new and active lean muscle mass helps us burn our fat stores and is the key to the effectiveness of Biocize.

Resistance

The amount of weight (load) or resistance the exerciser moves is another very important variable on Biocize. The higher the resistance, the less time and fewer repetitions we can tolerate, but the closer we come to a maximum voluntary contraction, commonly referred to as a maximum effort.

Maximum voluntary contractions involve the maximum amount of muscle *motor units* and greatly influence the hormonal benefit that is key to positive effects. In some exercise programs, a moderate weight is used for several repetitions. During the final few repetitions, the exercise begins to get quite difficult and could be considered a maximum voluntary contraction.

It is important to choose a resistance that allows you to progressively fatigue the muscle in the final few repetitions. This will promote the positive hormonal response induced by the exercise and will also trigger the muscles to adapt to increase their *cellular metabolism* and their *cross-sectional area*. In other words, they get larger, and therefore require more calories of energy, which causes greater fat loss.

Research shows that moderate to heavy resistance is more effective than low to moderate resistance when it comes to increasing testosterone, IGF-1, and human growth hormone. In your war on fat, you want to maximize this hormonal cascade. The increase in these hormones allows for an increase in many functions that help reduce fat stores and increase lean muscles mass.

Considerations for the Beginner

When you first choose a resistance, your goal is to learn the movement involved in the exercise. If you choose a resistance that is too great, you will likely perform the movement improperly. This will slow your success and could cause injury.

The repetitions are often higher in the beginning so you can teach your nervous system how to control the resistance. This is one of the reasons the first 45-Day Fat Wars Program was and still is so effective.

Considerations for More Advanced Exercisers (Phase 3 Programs)

As you make your way through the various programs, you will notice that the number of repetitions decreases while the resistance increases. This is in an attempt to make each repetition closer to a *maximum voluntary contraction*. You see, as a beginner you are learning the movement as you retrain your nervous system to perform better. Because your load is very low, it is only during the last few repetitions that you approach a maximum voluntary contraction. With fewer repetitions and higher resistance, you come closer to a maximum effort right from the first repetition! Your body can adjust to the higher stress load, and you will have enhanced metabolic adaptation for greater gains in muscle mass, strength, and a higher metabolic rate.

Drop Sets

The term *drop sets* refers to pausing (very briefly) during a set to lower the resistance you are using or to increase the help you are getting to perform the movement.

As an example:

You perform the dumbbell chest press with 15-pound dumbbells, attempting eight repetitions. After four repetitions, you pause briefly to switch to 10-pound dumbbells, then you complete the final four repetitions. The first four repetitions were near-maximum efforts, which fatigued you so you could not lift the 15 pounds. By switching to a lighter weight, you were able to perform four more repetitions, once again, a near-maximum effort.

If you chose 12-pound dumbbells for eight repetitions, you would need five much easier repetitions before the exercise became difficult. The initial repetitions serve little other than to tire you out! The total work accomplished is ultimately less—four reps at 15 pounds and four reps at 10 pounds makes 100 pounds. Eight reps at 12 pounds equals only 96 pounds. As you can see, the Fat Wars program is designed to give you the greatest effect in the least amount of time.

Rest between Sets

How long we rest between sets is also a very important variable in Biocize. During the resting phase, your muscles will attempt to replenish your intracellular energy stores (often called substrate stores). The length of time you rest will determine whether you completely replenish these stores.

The amount of time you rest between sets represents a balance between complete recovery and very little recovery. A growing body of research indicates that *partial recovery* between sets will have the greatest benefit for fat loss. This is likely because too much rest diminishes the *metabolic cost* of the exercise (not to mention making the workouts too long!), and too little rest doesn't allow us to perform high-quality repetitions that are near-maximum voluntary contractions. The name of the game here is to get in, accomplish what you came for, and get out. If you want to socialize, that's up to you, but realize the longer you stay in the gym, the fewer the results. Less equals more!

A 1998 study published in the *Journal of Strength and Conditioning Research* by Drs. Loebel and Kraemer proved that shorter rest periods led to increased post-workout testosterone levels. These increases in testosterone cause greater increases in lean muscle mass along with enhanced fat-burning potential.

FAT WARS PHASE I PROGRAM

EXERCISE OUTLINE FOR WEEKS 1-3

STRENGTH WORKOUT PROGRAM

Exercises	Sets	Repetitions	Tempo	Rest between sets
Ball squat on wall	2	8	3 descent 2 ascent	1:00
Hamstring curl with ball or machine cable curl	2	8	2 inwards 3 out	1:00
One armed row	2	8	2 ascent 3 descent	1:00
Dumbbell bench press	2	8	2 ascent 3 descent	1:00
Side lateral raise	2	8	2 ascent 3 descent	1:00
Biceps curls	2	8	2 ascent 3 descent	1:00
Overhead triceps extensions	2	8	2 ascent 3 descent	1:00

Core and abdominal exercises	Sets	Time under tension	Tempo	Rest between sets
Lower abdominal leg raise	2	60 seconds	Very slow	1:00
Superman	2	45 seconds	5-second holds	45 seconds
Abdominal crunch on ball	2	30 seconds	Slow descent Steady ascent	1:00

STRENGTH WORKOUT PROGRAM

WEEKS 4-6, PHASE I

Exercises	Sets	Repetitions	Tempo	Rest between sets
Ball squat on wall using dumbbell	2	7	4 down 2 up	1:00
Hamstring curl with ball or machine cable curl	2	7	2 inwards 4 out	1:00
One armed row	2	7	2 up 4 down	1:00
Dumbbell bench press	2	7	2 up 4 down	1:00
Dumbbell front raises, thumbs up	2	7	2 up 4 down	1:00
Biceps curls	2	7	2 up 4 down	1:00
Triceps extensions	2	7	2 to extend 4 to lower	1:00

Core and abdominal exercises	Sets	Reps	Tempo	Rest between sets
Lower abdominal activation from standing	2	60 seconds	Slow and controlled	1:00
Wall posture	2	45 seconds	Slow and controlled	1:00
Abdominal crunch on Swiss ball	2	6	2 up 4 down	1:00

SAMPLE WEEKLY EXERCISE SCHEDULE FOR PHASE I

Monday	Tuesday	Wednesday	Thursday	Friday	Weekend
Resistance Workout	Continuous Activity	Resistance Workout	Continuous Activity	Resistance Workout	Recreational Activities
Followed by 20-minute brisk walk	30-40 minutes	Followed by 20-minute brisk walk	30-40 minutes	Followed by 20-minute brisk walk	

FAT WARS PHASE II PROGRAM

EXERCISE OUTLINE FOR WEEKS 1-3

Strength Workout

Exercises	Sets	Repetitions	Tempo	Rest between sets
Sumo dumbbell squatft	2	8	4 descent 2 ascent	1:00
Hamstring curl with ball or machine cable curl	2	8	2 inward 4 out	1:00
Shoulder press	2	8	2 ascent 4 descent	1:00

Exercises	Sets	Repetitions	Tempo	Rest between sets
Modified pull-up	2	8	2 ascent 4 descent	1:00
Dumbbell or barbell bench press	2	8	2 ascent 4 descent	1:00
One-armed row	2	8	2 ascent 4 descent	1:00
Biceps curls	2	8	2 ascent 4 descent	1:00
Triceps extensions	2	8	2 ascent 4 descent	1:00

Core and abdominal exercises	Sets	Time under tension	Tempo	Rest between sets
Lower abdominal leg raise	2	60 seconds	Very slow	1:00
Superman	2	45 seconds	5-second holds	45 seconds
Abdominal crunch on ball	2	30 seconds	Slow descent Steady ascent	1:00

EXERCISE OUTLINE FOR WEEKS 4-6, PHASE II

Strength Workout

Exercises	Sets	Repetitions	Tempo	Rest between sets
Sumo dumbbell squat	2	7	5 descent 2 ascent	1:00
Hamstring curl with ball or machine cable curl	2	7	2 inward 5 out	1:00

Exercises	Sets	Repetitions	Tempo	Rest between sets
Shoulder press	2	7	2 ascent 5 descent	1:00
Modified pull-up	2	7	2 ascent 5 descent	1:00
Dumbbell or barbell bench press	2	7	2 ascent 5 descent	1:00
One-armed row	2	7	2 ascent 5 descent	1:00
Triceps extensions	2	7	2 ascent 5 descent	1:00

Core and abdominal exercises	Sets	Time under tension	Tempo	Rest between sets
Lower abdominal leg raise	2	60 seconds	Very slow	1:00
Superman	2	45 seconds	5-second holds	45 seconds
Abdominal crunch on ball	2	30 seconds	Slow descent Steady ascent	1:00

SAMPLE WEEKLY EXERCISE SCHEDULE FOR PHASE II

Monday	Tuesday	Wednesday	Thursday	Friday	Weekend
Resistance Workout	Continuous Activity	Resistance Workout	Continuous Activity	Resistance Workout	Recreational Activities
Followed by 20-minute brisk walk	40-50 minutes	Followed by 20-minute brisk walk	40-50 minutes	Followed by 20-minute brisk walk	

FAT WARS PHASE III PROGRAM

EXERCISE OUTLINE FOR WEEKS 1-3

Workout #1

Exercises	Sets	Repetitions	Tempo	Rest between sets
Dumbbell lunges	3	6 each leg	2 descent 2 ascent	1:00
Ball hamstring curls or machine cable curls	3	6	3 ascent 5 descent	1:00
Pull-ups (assisted if necessary)	3	6	3 ascent 5 descent	1:00
Bent over row or hanging row	3	6	3 ascent 5 descent	1:00
Biceps curls	3	6	3 ascent 5 descent	1:00

Core and abdominal exercises	Sets	Time under tension	Tempo	Rest between sets
Roll-out	2	60 seconds	Very slow	1:00
Superman	2	45 seconds	5-second holds	45 seconds
Abdominal crunch on ball	2	30 seconds	Slow descent Steady ascent	1:00

Workout #2

Exercises	Sets	Repetitions	Tempo	Rest between sets
Barbell front squat	3	6	5 down 3 up	1:00
Dead lift	3	6	1 up 2 down	1:00
Dumbbell or barbell bench press	3	6	3 up 5 down	1:00
Shoulder press	3	6	3 up 5 down	1:00
Triceps push-up	3	6	3 ascent 5 descent	1:00

Shoulder stability activities	Sets	Repetitions	Tempo	Rest between sets
Rotator cuff internal rotation	2	6	3 up 5 down	1:00
Rotator cuff external rotation	2	6	3 up 5 down	1:00
Side raise to 45 degrees	2	6	3 up 5 down	1:00

EXERCISE OUTLINE FOR WEEKS 4-6

Workout #1

Exercises	Sets	Repetitions	Tempo	Rest between sets
Dumbbell lunges	3	5 each leg	3 down 3 up	1:00
Romanian dead lift	3	6	3 up 6 down	1:00
Chin-ups	3	6	3 up 6 down	1:00
Bent over row or hanging row	3	6	3 up 6 down	1:00
Biceps curls	4	6	3 up 6 down	1:00

Core and abdominal exercises	Sets	Time under tension	Tempo	Rest between sets
Roll-out	3	90 seconds	Very slow	1:00
Wood chop	3	60 seconds	5-second holds	45 seconds
Abdominal crunch on ball	3	30 seconds	Very slow	1:00

Workout #2

Exercises	Sets	Repetitions	Tempo	Rest between sets
Dead lift	3	8	1 up 2 down	1:00
Barbell front squat	3	6	6 down 3 up	1:00
Dumbbell or barbell bench press, Incline	3	6	3 up 6 down	1:00
Shoulder press	3	6	3 up 6 down	1:00
Triceps push-up	4	6	3 ascent 6 descent	1:00

Shoulder stability activities	Sets	Repetitions	Tempo	Rest between sets
Rotator cuff internal rotation	2	6	3 up 6 down	1:00
Rotator cuff external rotation	2	6	3 up 6 down	1:00
Side raise to 45 degrees	2	6	3 up 6 down	1:00

SAMPLE WEEKLY EXERCISE SCHEDULE FOR PHASE III

Monday	Tuesday	Wednesday	Thursday	Friday	Weekend
Resistance Workout #1	Resistance Workout #2	Continuous Activity	Resistance Workout #3	Resistance Workout #4	Recreational Activities
Followed by 20-minute brisk walk		50-60 minutes	Followed by 20-minute brisk walk		

EXERCISE DESCRIPTIONS

Chest Section

Barbell Bench Press

Begin with the barbell positioned above the top of your chest, with your arms outstretched (you may want assistance taking the bar off the barbell rack). Lower the barbell in a moderate and consistent arc toward the bottom of your chest. As you will note from the photo, the elbows do not point straight out to the sides; they are positioned out and down slightly toward your feet.

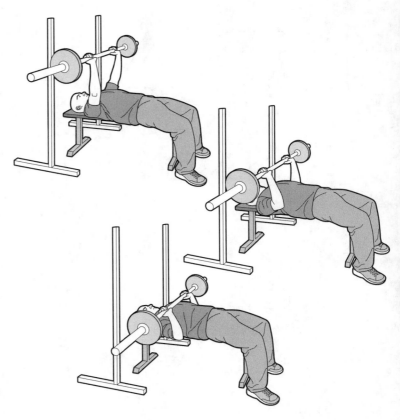

When the bar makes contact with your chest, pause, then return to the start position by following the same pattern. The motion should feel natural. If it doesn't at first, try practising the motion in a mirror while standing.

Before lowering the barbell, inhale partially, hold your breath, and tighten your abdominals slightly by drawing in your belly button. As you press upward, exhale steadily through pursed lips.

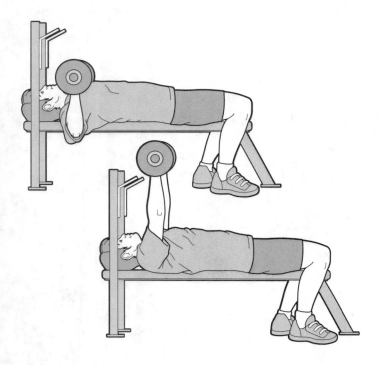

Dumbbell Bench Press

Lie flat on a bench with dumbbells to the sides of your chest and with your elbows directly under your hands. Press up and together, and return to start position.

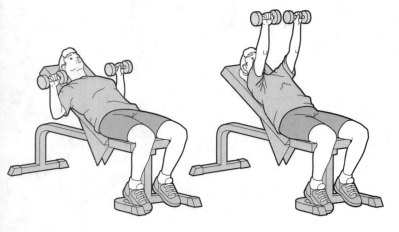

Incline Dumbbell Bench Press

Using a bench that adjusts to a 45-degree angle, begin with the dumbbells beside your chest with the elbows directly under your hands. Press up and together, and return to start position.

Shoulder Section

Shoulder Press

Begin with the dumbbells positioned parallel to your ears, with the elbows directly below the dumbbells. Press upward and together until your arms are fully outstretched. Pause, and return to start position.

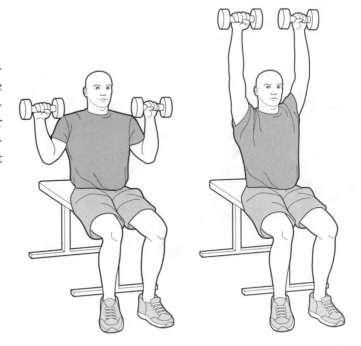

Rotator Cuff Internal Rotation

Lay on your side on a bench, grasping a dumbbell in the hand that is near the floor. With your elbow bent to 90 degrees, rotate the dumbbell up and in toward your torso. Pause, and return.

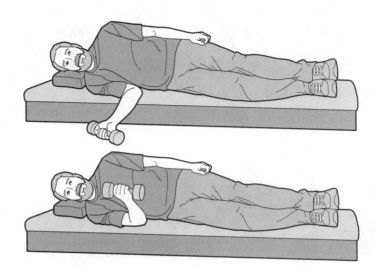

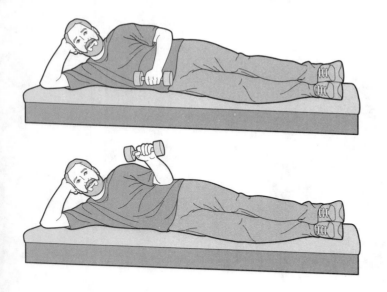

Rotator Cuff External Rotation

Lay on your side on a bench, grasping a dumbbell in the hand that is on the side facing up. With your elbow bent to 90 degrees, rotate the dumbbell up until it is vertical. Pause, and return.

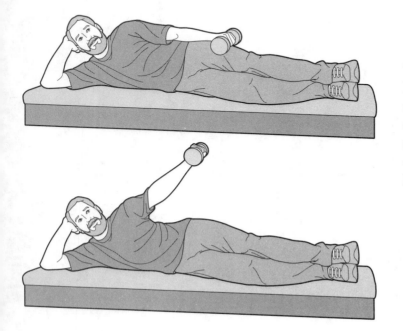

Side Raise to 45 Degrees

Lay on your side with the arm on the upward side outstretched and clasping the dumbbell. Raise your arm up until your arm is at a 45-degree angle to your body. Pause here, and return.

Lateral Raises

Stand up straight with a dumbbell in each hand at your sides. Raise the dumbbells at your side until they are parallel to your shoulders. Keep your thumbs pointing forward (not down). Pause at the top position, and return.

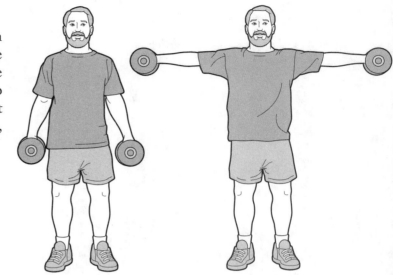

Leg Section

Front Squat

Cross your arms over the barbell, with your shoulders supporting the bar. Inhale partially and hold, and draw your belly button in to tighten your abdominals slightly. Descend by dropping your hips and flexing at the knee, until the back of your upper leg (hamstrings) contacts the back of your lower leg. Pause and return to start position, breathing out steadily as you ascend.

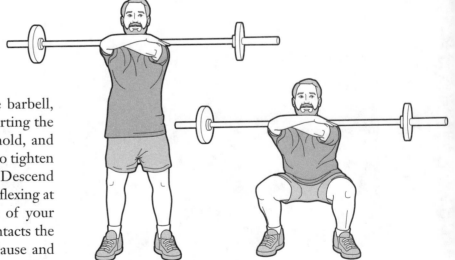

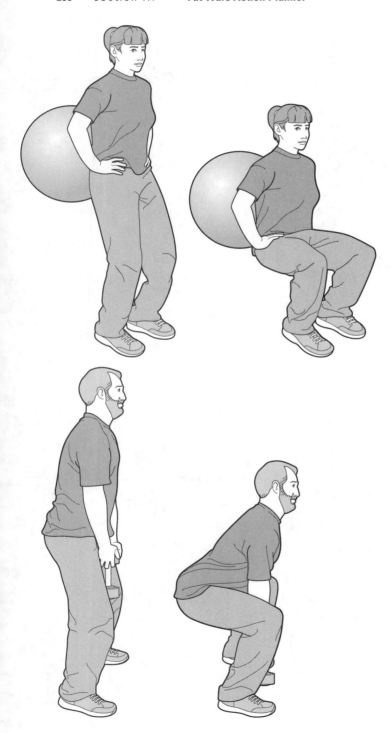

Ball Squat on Wall

With the Swiss ball placed between the wall and your tailbone, stand with your chest up and facing forward. Your feet should be out and away slightly, with toes pointed forward. Drop your hips and flex at the knee to descend, pause, and extend up and back to start position. Do not lean back into the ball, and do not roll your torso forward as you ascend. Keep your abdominals tight throughout, breathing out as you ascend.

Sumo Squat

Stand with a hip-width stance, holding a dumbbell between your legs with both hands. Tighten your abdomen by drawing in your navel and holding your breath. Lower by flexing at the knee and extending your hips backward. Pause when your thigh is parallel to the floor, then return.

Dumbbell Lunge

Grab an appropriately weighted dumbbell in each hand. Stand with both feet together. Step forward and slowly drop your hips down until the knee of your back leg is only a few inches from the floor. Pause, and return to start position by pushing off your front leg and using pressure to pull forward with your back leg. Repeat with the other leg for the suggested amount of repetitions.

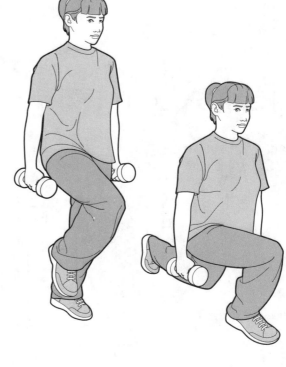

Hamstring Curl with Ball

Place your feet on the ball as illustrated, and raise your back up and off of the floor. (This, at first, will be difficult, as the ball is unbalanced. With a little practise, it will become quite easy.) Bring the ball in toward your body and raise the hips simultaneously. Once you've brought the ball in as far as you can, pause, and move the ball back out steadily.

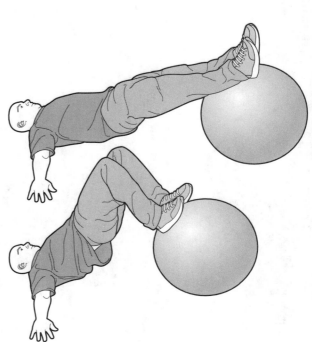

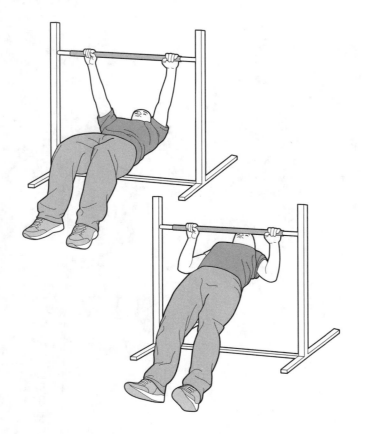

Back Section

Hanging Row

Place a barbell across a squat rack (in a gym) or use a bar that is secured firmly on two supports. Grasp the bar so your arms are slightly wider apart than shoulder width, and place your feet out and away from your body. You should be hanging off the bar. Pull your chest up toward the bar, pause, then return slowly to start position.

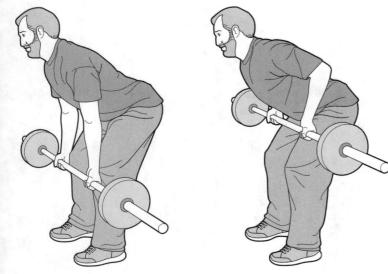

Bent Over Row

Grasp a barbell or dumbbells, and soften your knees into a slight bend. Bend over at the hips (not at the waist) while keeping your back in a neutral curve. Keep your abdominals relatively tight to support your back.

Draw the barbell upward and in toward your navel, where you will pause, then return to the start position. Keep the bar close to your body throughout the movement to reduce the stress on your lower back.

Dead Lift

With the barbell on the floor, place your shins near the bar, drop your hips down (maintaining a neutral curve in the back), and bend your knees until you can grasp the bar with your arms on the outside of your legs. Make sure your back is not rounded. Look forward.

To ascend, breathe in partially, and hold. Draw your belly button inward. Extend your legs and hips, focusing on keeping your back in its neutral curve while you move your hips forward. As you are extending and moving upward, breathe out steadily.

To descend, repeat the breathing pattern by holding your breathe at the top and exhaling only when the barbell touches the ground again.

Modified Pull-up

As with the hanging row, place a barbell across the squat rack. This time it should be near shoulder height. Hang from the bar with your feet just ahead of your hips.

To begin, pull yourself upward until your collarbone reaches the bar. Pause, and return.

As you will note, your legs may assist you in this exercise, but it is an upper body exercise. Only use the minimum amount of help from the legs.

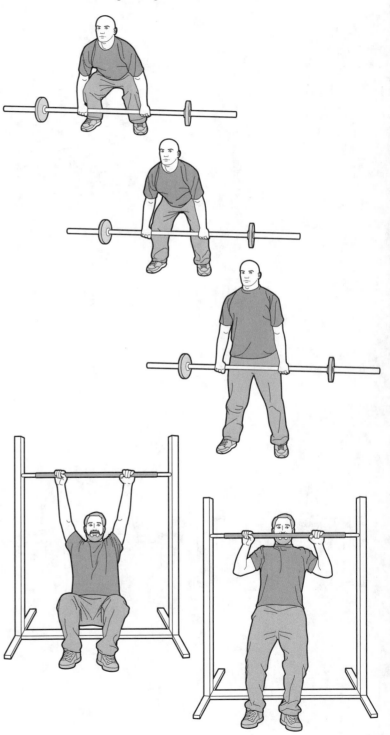

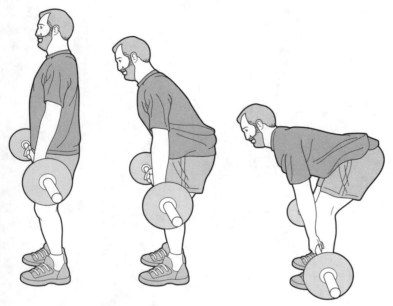

Romanian Dead Lift

Grasp the bar as shown in the illustration. One palm should face forward, the other palm should face back. Hold your breath for a moment and tighten your abdominals as you descend, bending only at the hip (not the waist). Keep your back in its neutral curve, and maintain a short distance between the bar and your body.

Move down until your hamstrings tighten, pause, then move back up while breathing out.

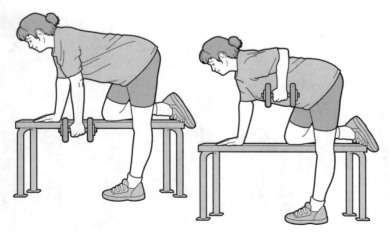

One Armed Row

Place one hand and one shin on the bench, with the opposite leg on the floor. Your other hand should be grasping the dumbbell. Your arm should be hanging straight down from your shoulder. Draw the dumbbell up and slightly back toward your belt line as if you are starting a lawn mower. Pause at the top position, and lower.

Abdominal Section

Wood Chop
(can be done with tubing as well as with cable system)

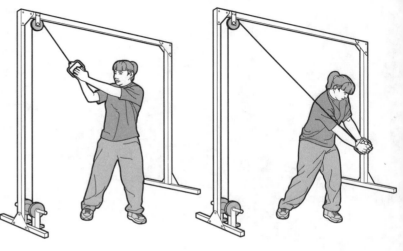

Stand perpendicular to the cable apparatus. Grasp handle. Make sure the hand closest to the cable has the palm facing forward, with the other hand overlapping. Before moving, tighten your abdominals by drawing your navel inward. Rotate cable across your body and down, with your arms outstretched. Concentrate on using your abdominals to perform the motion.

To return, slowly counter rotate until you reach the start position again.

Roll-out

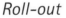

Place the Swiss ball in front of you and lean onto it with your knees, hips, and shoulders in a straight line. Your elbows and forearms should be on the ball. Inhale partially, hold, and draw your navel inward. Slowly move your arms out and away from your body. Pause, and return, breathing out as you do.

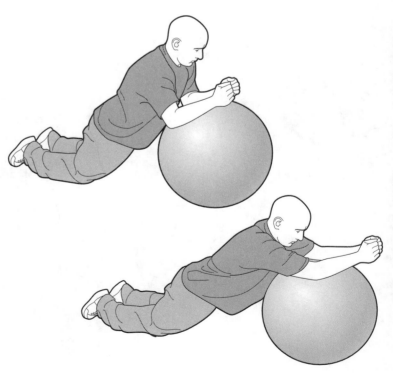

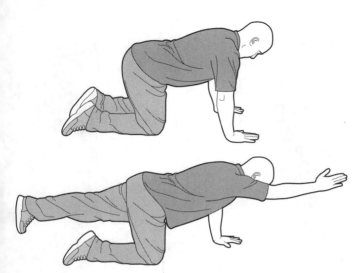

Superman

Get on the floor in an all-fours position. Be sure to keep your back relatively flat (neutral spine) Extend your right leg and your left arm, hold for a count of 5 seconds, and return. Repeat with the opposite limbs.

When you extend, try to keep the spine from rotating or rounding.

Abdominal Crunches on Ball

Start from a seated position and lower your body slowly by moving your feet away from the ball. As you are moving your feet, progressively place more of your back onto the ball. When the ball is supported under your lower back, you are in the correct start position.

From here, start the exercise by drawing your belly button toward your spine and extend backward until your shoulder blades and head rest on the ball. You are wrapped around the ball. Now slowly and steadily curl up from the head and upper torso, flexing forward until you are almost vertical. Slowly reverse the curl and return to start position.

While performing this exercise, keep your tongue on the roof of your mouth, behind your front teeth. This stabilizes the neck muscles to support you better.

Lower Abdominal Leg Raises

Lie on the floor with the soles of your feel on the ground and knees flexed. Place your hands under your lower back. Inhale partially and hold. Draw your belly button in toward your spine. Flex your leg at the hip and bring your knee toward your chest slightly, then lower and extend out and away from you, breathing out slowly as you do. When your foot is fully extended and touching the ground, relax your abdominals and return your leg to its starting position. Begin again with the opposite leg.

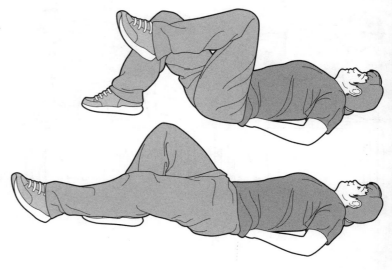

Arm Section

Biceps Curls

Stand up straight with a dumbbell in each hand in the front of your thighs, palms forward. Flex up at the elbow to raise the dumbbells, pause at the top, and lower.

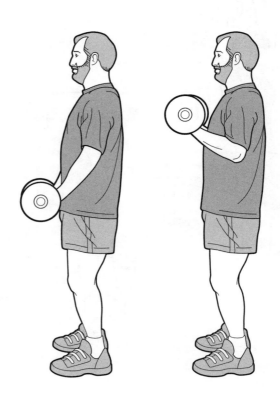

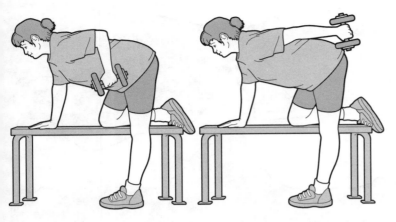

Triceps Extension

Stand as in the one-armed row, then raise your elbow until it is flush with your torso. Extend your forearm at the elbow fully, pause, and return.

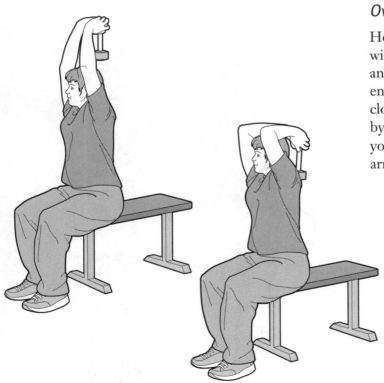

Overhead Triceps Extension

Hold a dumbbell over your head with both hands around the handle, and wrap your fingers around the ends. Your elbows should be very close together. Lower the dumbbell by flexing at the elbow, but keep your elbows stationary. Extend your arms up to return.

appendix

FAT WARS SUPPLEMENT RECOMMENDATIONS

Throughout Section I of this book I mention nutrients that offer special benefits in the Fat Wars. Below, supplement suggestions are listed by chapter for easy reference.

In my many years in the health industry, I have come to realize that there are only a handful of respectable and trustworthy product manufacturers. The recommendations I present here are, to the best of my knowledge, some of the top products in the industry.

Note: All the recommended supplements in this section can be found throughout Canada at local health food retailers and selected supermarket and pharmacy chains.

As Seen In Chapter 1:

In this chapter I explained the fat-loss benefits of creating extra heat through the process referred to as thermogenesis. As thermogenesis takes place, the body enhances its fat-burning ability. Thermogenesis occurs when we eat (diet-induced thermogenesis, in which protein has the highest thermogenic value), when we exercise (physical thermogenesis), and when we are trying to keep warm (shivering thermogenesis). But thermogenesis can also be increased through supplementation of thermogenic nutrients.

Two key nutrients that show promise in enhancing this thermic effect are *Citrus aurantium* and green tea extract. Both thermogenic nutrients can be found individually as supplements in your local health food store or in specially designed formulas that combine them (along with other nutrients). Most natural substances work even better when combined in a synergistic formulation. While there are a number of fat-burning nutrients listed individually, you don't have to hunt each of them down. Many can be found in combination with other fat-burning nutrients in two special formulas listed below. Both formulas target a variety of biochemical problems inherent to weight loss, including thermogenesis through the activation of the enzymes and messengers necessary for fat loss.

lean+:

- increases the breakdown of stored fat (lipolysis) by activating fat-releasing enzymes and increasing intracellular communication;

- increases the metabolic rate by increasing thermogenesis (body heat production) and stimulating the thyroid;

- curbs excess appetite;

- improves the metabolism of carbohydrates (sugars) so fewer will convert to fat;

- inhibits excess production of fat;

- increases energy;

- lowers LDL and VLDL (bad) cholesterol levels while increasing HDL (good) cholesterol levels;

- protects against damage by free radicals.

lean+ (with green tea extract and *Citrus aurantium*)
Manufactured for:
ehn inc. (greens+)

317 Adelaide Street West, Suite 501
Toronto, Ontario • M5V 1P9
Tel: 416-977-3505 • Toll-free: 877-500-7888
Fax: 416-977-4184 • Web site: www.greenspluscanada.com

abs+ (with standardized (high EGCG) green tea extract and CLA)
Manufactured for:
ehn inc. (greens+)
317 Adelaide Street West, Suite 501
Toronto, Ontario • M5V 1P9
Tel: 416-977-3505 • Toll-free: 877-500-7888
Fax: 416-977-4184 • Web site: www.greenspluscanada.com

As Seen In Chapter 3:

In this chapter I spoke about the numerous daily cravings people deal
with that quickly bring a halt to success in the Fat Wars. I also mentioned natural ways to deal with these insatiable cravings through
nutrient intervention. One way to accomplish this is to consume high
alphalactalbumin whey-protein isolates that also have high GMPs.
The extremely high tryptophan content will help raise serotonin levels in the brain (cutting off cravings neurochemicaly), and the GMPs
will stimulate the hormone CCK—responsible for satiety. The other
way is to consume anti-craving nutrients in synergistic formulations.
Both are listed below.

High alpha whey-protein isolate
(found in proteins+ and transform+)

High alphalactalbumin whey isolates are produced using a patented isolation process that creates the highest biological value of any protein on
the market today. High-alphalactalbumin whey isolates contain two and
a half times the cysteine levels present in other whey-protein isolates,
making them an excellent and unsurpassed source of natural glutathione
builders (which raise overall immune status).

The levels of the amino acid tryptophan in high-alphalactalbumin
whey isolates are triple those of other whey-protein isolates. Tryptophan

is needed by the body to produce the neurotransmitter serotonin. Extensive research over the past forty years has established that the activity level of serotonin has a material impact on levels of insomnia, pain sensitivity, anxiety, and depression. Serotonin has also been demonstrated to have appetite-suppressant qualities.

High alphalactalbumin whey isolates also contain the highest levels of glycomacropeptides (GMPs) found in any whey-protein product. GMPs are powerful stimulators of a hormone called cholecystokinin (CCK), which plays many essential roles in our gastrointestinal system. CCK stimulates the release of enzymes from the pancreas and increases gall-bladder contraction and bowel motility. One of CCK's most incredible properties is its ability to regulate our food intake by sending satiation signals to the brain, making it a potential diet aid. In animal studies, a rise in CCK is always followed by a large reduction in food intake. In human studies, whey-protein glycomacropeptides were shown to increase CCK production by 415% within 20 minutes after ingestion.

High-alphalactalbumin proteins+ and transform+ are manufactured in Canada for:
ehn inc. (greens+)
317 Adelaide Street West, Suite 501
Toronto, Ontario • M5V 1P9
Tel: 416-977-3505 • Toll-free: 877-500-7888
Fax: 416-977-4184 • Web site: www.greenspluscanada.com

Anti-Craving Formulas
(crave free)

Many people cannot fight their physiological urge to binge eat, especially where insulin-spiking carbohydrates are concerned. It is important to recognize that in many cases the failure to lose your excess fat may be due to various biochemical imbalances in brain chemicals that drive you to eat excessively. It is sometimes almost impossible to ignore the insatiable cravings for these foods, and when we finally give in we feel a great wave of relief that unfortunately lasts only a little while and leaves us with another pound or two.

In Chapter 3, I covered the various aspects of the brain chemical serotonin and how it affects the craving and award centers of your brain. But serotonin is not alone when it comes to cravings-curbing brain chemicals. Certain nutrients have been shown to help overcome insatiable cravings by modulating these brain chemicals (mostly serotonin and dopamine). You can find these natural nutrients in the synergistic formulation (crave-free) presented below.

Warning: Those taking selective serotonin reuptake inhibitors, tricyclic antidepressants, or monoamine oxidase inhibitors should consult a health-care professional before taking these products.

crave-free is manufactured in Canada for:
ehn inc. (greens+)
317 Adelaide Street West, Suite 501
Toronto, Ontario • M5V 1P9
Tel: 416-977-3505 • Toll-free: 877-500-7888
Fax: 416-977-4184 • Web site: www.greenspluscanada.com

As Seen In Chapter 4:

In this chapter I spoke about nature's way to higher HGH levels through natural substances such as colostrum and amino-acid secretagogues. These substances may be one of the safest and best ways to achieve higher HGH levels in the body naturally. Recommendations follow.

Colostrum

Colostrum is the pre-milk substance produced by female mammals prior to giving birth. Colostrum contains specialized immune factors as well as growth factors. These powerful components (as well as others) work to enhance overall immunity, health, and well-being; they build muscle and burn body fat, increase energy, improve memory, and improve overall mood. These bovine colostrum factors are identical in molecular formation to human colostrum and therefore easily transferrable from one species (cow) to another (human).

The nutrient L-carnitine is a very powerful ally in the Fat Wars. Carnitine helps transport fatty acids into the furnaces (mitochondria) of our cells so that they can be incinerated. L-carnitine is presently restricted in Canada; however, it is concentrated in colostrum, and supplementing with bovine colostrum may be a great way to increase natural carnitine levels.

The earlier the colostrum is taken from the source, the more potent it is. Studies show that colostrum harvested 12 hours after birth contains only one-third of the immune and growth factors present in colostrum taken at birth.

For maximum potency and bioactivity, look for colostrum harvested from select Grade A dairy cows within the first 6 hours, processed in a certified GMP (Good Manufacturing Practices) facility under the strictest of quality standards using very low heat. The product that meets this criteria is marketed in Canada by:

Sequel Naturals
Toll-free: 1-866-839-8863
e-mail: info@sequelnaturals.com • Web site: www.sequelnaturals.com

HGH Secretagogues

As mentioned in Chapter 4, HGH levels can be naturally elevated using specialized amino acid secretagogues. The one product I have reviewed that seems to contain all the amino acids necessary for effective HGH stimulation is SomaLife gHP by Soma Health Products Inc. You can contact the company toll-free at 1-877-256-7662.

As Seen In Chapter 5:

In this chapter I spoke about his fat and her fat and the biochemical difference in each as it pertained to the Fat Wars. There were mentions of stinging nettle (using an aqueous or methanol extraction) as well as a bioflavinoid called chrysin, the indoles I3C and DIM, and soy-protein isolates. Below are the recommended products as they are found.

Aqueous or Methanol Extracted Stinging Nettle (Urtica dioica)

As men age, their ratio of estrogen to testosterone increases partly due to an increase in the testosterone-binding protein-sex-hormone-binding globulin (SHBG). Stinging nettle has been shown to help free bound testosterone by competing for receptor sites on the SHBG molecule.

Aqueous extracted stinging nettle can be found:

In the product enact+
Manufactured in Canada for:
ehn inc. (greens+)
317 Adelaide Street West, Suite 501
Toronto, Ontario • M5V 1P9
Tel: 416-977-3505 • Toll-free: 877-500-7888
Fax: 416-977-4184 • Web site: www.greenspluscanada.com

Chrysin with Piperine Extract

As men age, a great deal of their testosterone is chemically converted into estrogen via the enzyme aromatase. One of the most powerful inhibitors of this conversion can be found in the natural bioflavonoid chrysin. Chrysin was shown to be similar in potency and effectiveness to the conversion-inhibiting drug aminoglutethimide. Chrysin has a poor absorption ability. To make it bioavailable to the body, an enhanced delivery ingredient such as piperine (black pepper extract) must accompany it.

Chrysin with piperine extract can be found:

In U.S.A.:
In the product His Fat Hormonal Equalizer for Men (with stinging nettle root, chrysin, and piperine extract)
Distributed by:
Transforming Health Inc.
Tel: 604-987-8733 • Toll-free: 1-866-FAT-AWAY (328-2929)
Fax: 604-987-8735 • Web site: www.fatwars.com

Soy Protein Isolates

Look for non-GMO soy protein isolate, which contains the highest-quality water-extracted soy protein on the market today. It has a biological value of 100, the same as an egg when it comes to protein quality. The product transform+ uses only non-GMO soy protein isolate as its soy protein source.

In Canada:
transform+ (containing non-GMO soy isolate) is manufactured in Canada for:
ehn inc. (greens+)
317 Adelaide Street West, Suite 501
Toronto, Ontario • M5V 1P9
Tel: 416-977-3505 • Toll-free: 877-500-7888
Fax: 416-977-4184 • Web site: www.greenspluscanada.com

As Seen In Chapter 6:

In this chapter I spoke about macronutrients, protein, fats, and carbs, and made mention of a number of beneficial nutrients in the Fat Wars including whey protein, CLA, fish oil, and beta-glucan. Below are the recommended products they are found in.

Whey Protein

Whey is a by-product of the cheese-making process. Earlier products were referred to as whey concentrates. These contained as little as 30% to 40% dietary proteins but were filled with huge amounts of fat, lactose (milk sugar), and denatured (damaged) proteins.

The majority of the products available today come from newer processes—ion-exchange and cross-flow membrane extraction. They have a higher percentage of dietary proteins than their predecessors—high enough to merit the label "isolates."

The newest generation of whey isolates can contain more than 90% pure dietary proteins, with almost no dietary fats and minimal levels of lactose. They are also very expensive to produce. Because of the cost, many manufacturers tend to mix the isolates with less expensive concentrates and still call them isolates. Only a very small percentage of companies use 100% isolates. When you purchase whey isolate, look for the highest levels of the major protein fraction called alphalactalbumin. The alpha portion is the most bioavailable to the human body.

High alphalactalbumin proteins+ and transform+ are manufactured in Canada for:

ehn inc. (greens+)
317 Adelaide Street West, Suite 501
Toronto, Ontario • M5V 1P9
Tel: 416-977-3505 • Toll-free: 877-500-7888
Fax: 416-977-4184 • Web site: www.greenspluscanada.com

Conjugated Linoleic Acid (CLA)

CLA is a natural polyunsaturated fat found primarily in beef and milk. CLA has been shown over the years to have many beneficial effects on our physiology, some of which include potent antioxidant activity, anti-carcinogenic properties, anti-catabolic properties (stopping muscle wasting), powerful immune system-enhancing capabilities, and the reduction of body fat. Instead of burning fat directly, CLA may affect the rate at which fat cells grow.

CLA can be found in a synergistic combination with standardized (high EGCG) green tea extract in the product abs+. abs+ is manufactured in Canada for:
ehn inc. (greens+)
317 Adelaide Street West, Suite 501
Toronto, Ontario • M5V 1P9
Tel: 416-977-3505 • Toll-free: 877-500-7888
Fax: 416-977-4184 • Web site: www.greenspluscanada.com

Essential Fatty Acid (EFA)

Like vitamins, EFAs are essential to health. Older literature, in fact, refers to them as vitamin F. Our bodies cannot manufacture them, so they must be obtained from our diet. Referred to as omega-3 and omega-6, these friendly fats help keep insulin functioning properly, regulate oxygen and energy transport, help form red blood cells, keep hormone-producing glands active, help make joint lubricants, and in the right combinations also provide a fat-burning effect.

I highly recommend daily supplementation of oil from cold-water wild fish. The omega-3 fatty acids these special fats contain are in their pre-activated forms—meaning the body can use them very efficiently. Fish oil will go a long way to increasing your fat-burning efforts in the Fat Wars.

In Canada:

o3mega enteric-coated wild fish oil (sardines, anchovies, and mackerel)

Research (the *New England Journal of Medicine*, June 13, 1996) indicates that enteric-coated fish oils may present an enhanced method of delivery, especially for people with compromised gastrointestinal systems.

o3mega triple fish oil is manufactured in Canada for:
ehn inc. (greens+)
317 Adelaide Street West, Suite 501
Toronto, Ontario • M5V 1P9
Tel: 416-977-3505 • Toll-free: 877-500-7888
Fax: 416-977-4184 • Web site: www.greenspluscanada.com

Starch Blocker

Phaseolamin 2250

I recommend this product only for people who have a very difficult time staying away from the starchy carbs. It is also an excellent product to take on cheat days (as long as you don't overdo it). Phaseolamin 2250 (Phase 2) is the first clinically proven, standardized, all-natural supplement for neutralizing starch calories. In studies, 1 gram of Phaseolamin 2250 was shown to neutralize more than 500 grams of dietary starch— or more than 2,250 calories (of carbohydrate).

Phaseolamin 2250 and Phase 2 are registered trademarks of:
Pharmachem Laboratories Inc.
265 Harrison Ave., Kearny NJ USA 07032
Toll-free: (800)526-0609 • Web site: www.starchstopper.com.

Phaseolamin 2250 and Phase 2 are found in the product:
Fat Wars Ultimate Starch Stopper
Distributed by:
Transforming Health Inc.
Tel: 604-987-8733
Toll-free: 1-866-FAT-AWAY (328-2929) • Fax: 604-987-8735
Web site: www.fatwars.com

Oat Beta-glucans

Oat bran is one of the best sources of soluble fiber. The cardiovascular benefits, including cholesterol-lowering effects, of oat-soluble fiber are well documented in more than thirty peer-reviewed, published clinical studies. Oats also offer benefits for hypertension, diabetes, and obesity.

OatVantage oat bran concentrate (beta-glucan) is a registered trademark of:
Nurture Inc.
1600 Stout, Suite 710
Denver, CO 80202
Phone: 303-260-6920 • Fax: 303-260-6921
Web site: www.oatvantage.com

OatVantage oat bran concentrate is found in the product:
Fat Wars Ultimate Fiber Complex
Distributed by:
Transforming Health Inc.
Tel: 604-987-8733 • Toll-free: 1-866-FAT-AWAY (328-2929)
Fax: 604-987-8735 • Web site: www.fatwars.com

Grass-Fed Beef

According to a study in the journal *Animal Science* in 2000, grain-fed beef can have an omega-6 to omega-3 ratio higher than twenty to one. This kind of fatty-acid ratio is what disturbs our overall health balance (homeostasis) and leads to obesity and disease. Not only is grain-fed supermarket beef completely out of whack with nature in its overall fatty-acid profile, but the majority of the beef cuts available also have an overall high fat content, ranging from 35% to 75%, with most of it coming from saturated fat.

On the other hand, grass-fed beef offers an omega-6 to omega-3 ratio of three to one, which is the ideal ratio for a healthy diet (and the same ratio fish offers). The other major benefit of grass-fed beef is that less than 10% of its fat is saturated. It also offers a very good supply of natural CLA. For these and many more reasons outlined on the Fat Wars Web site (www.fatwars.com) I highly recommend grass-fed beef over grain-fed. Below are recommended suppliers.

Bar 7 Ranch
PO Box 1942
Vanderhoof, BC • V0J 3A0
Tel: (250) 567-2860 • e-mail info@bar7ranch.ca
Web site: www.bar7ranch.ca

As Seen In Section II:

Recommended organic products (most are available nationwide) listed by subject:

Organic whole sprouted grains
Silver Hills Bakery
PO Box 2250,
Abbotsford, BC • V2T 4X2
Tel: 604-850-5600 • Fax: 604- 856-5689
e-mail info@silverhillsbakery.ca • Web site: www.silverhillsbakery.com

Natural stone-ground whole-grain cereals and flours
Bob's Red Mill Natural Foods
5209 SE International Way
Milwaukie, OR 97222
Toll free: 1-800-349-2173 • Fax: 503-653-1339
Web site: www.bobsredmill.com

Organic packaged salad mixes
Earthbound farm
1721 San Juan Highway
San Juan Bautista, CA 95045
Toll-free: 1-800-690-3200 • e-mail: info@ebfarm.com

Organic milk, cream, butter, yogurt, cheese, and sour cream
Organic Meadow
OntarBio Organic Farmers' Co-operative
RR# 5 • Guelph, Ontario • N1H 6J2
Tel: 519-767-9694
e-mail: info@ontarbio.com • Web site: www.ontarbio.com

Milk, cheese, butter, cream cheese, cottage cheese, sour cream, and cream
Organic Valley
La Farge, WI 54639
Tel: 608-625-2600
Web site: www.organicvalley.com

Frozen yogurt, ice cream
Stonyfield Farms
Londonderry, NH,
Toll-free: 1-800-PRO-COWS (776-2697)
Tel: 603-437-4040
Web site: www.stonyfield.com

Cascadian Farm
Sedro-Wooley, WA 98284
Toll-free: 1-800-624-4123

Organic goat milk, cheese, and yogurt
McLennan Creek Dairy Ltd.
30854 Olund Road
Abbotsford, BC • V4X 1Z9
Tel: 1-888-668-4823
e-mail: glenacres@rslnet.net
Web site: www.organicgoatcheese.ca

Vegetarian alternatives
Yves Veggie Cuisine
1638 Derwent Way
Delta, BC • V3M 6R9
Toll-free: 1-800-667-9837
Web site: www.yvesveggie.com

Note: Look for updated information on products, exercises, and research on the Fat Wars Web site at www.fatwars.com.

For United States residents, please visit www.fatwars.com to order American Fat Wars products on-line.

REFERENCES

Introduction

1. Atkins, R. *Dr. Atkins' New Diet Revolution*. New York: M. Evans, 1999.

2. Bland, J., and S.H. Benum. *Genetic Nutritioneering*: Keats Publishing, 1999.

3. Challem, J., B. Berkson, and M.D. Smith. *Syndrome X: The Complete Nutritional Program to Prevent and Reverse Insulin Resistance*. New York: John Wiley & Sons, 2000.

4. Colditz, G.A. "Economic costs of obesity." *Am J Clin Nutr* [spell out name of journal] 55 (1992): 503-507s.

5. Graci, S. *The Food Connection*. Toronto: Macmillan, 2001.

6. King, B. J. *Fat Wars: 45 Days to Transform Your Body*. Toronto: Macmillan, 2002.

7. Masuno, H., et al. "Bisphenol A in combination with insulin can accelerate the conversion of 3T3-L1 fibroblasts to adipocytes." *J lipid Res* [spell out name of journal] 3 (2002): 676-684.

8. National Institutes of Health (NIH) News Release: First Federal Obesity Clinical Guidelines Released, June 17, 1998.

9. Sturm, R., and K.B. Wells. "Does Obesity Contribute as Much to Morbidity as Poverty or Smoking?" Public Health 115 (2001): 229-295.

Chapter 1

Astrup, A., C. Lundsgaard, J. Madsen, and N. Christiensen. "Enhanced thermogenic responsiveness during chronic ephedrine treatment in man." *Journal of Clinical Nutrition* 42 (1985): 83-94.

Astrup, A. "Pharmacology of thermogenic drugs." *American Journal of Clinical Nutrition* 55 (1992): 246S-249S

Barenys, M., et al. "Effect of Exercise and Protein Intake on Energy Expenditure in Adolescents." *Rev Esp Fisiol* 49:4 (1993): 209-217.

Cassidy, C.M. "Nutrition and Health in Agriculturists and Hunter-Gatherers: A Case Study of Two Prehistoric Populations." Nutritional Anthropology Pleasantville, New York: 117-145.

Collins, S., et al. "Strain Specific Response to Beta-3 Adrenergic Receptor Agonist Treatment of Diet Induced Obesity in Mice." *Endocrinol* 138 (1997): 405-413.

Daly, P.A. et al. "Ephedrine, caffeine and aspirin: safety and efficacy for treatment of human obesity." *International Journal of Obesity* 17.

Dulloo A., et al. "Efficacy of a Green Tea Extract Rich in Catechin Polyphenols and Caffeine in Increasing 24-h Energy Expenditure and Fat Oxidation in Humans." *American Journal of Clinical Nutrition* 70 (1999): 1040-1045.

Dulloo, A.G., J. Seydoux, L. Girardier, et al. "Green Tea and Thermogenesis: Interactions between Catechin-Polyphenols, Caffeine, and Sympathetic Activity." *American Journal of Clinical Nutrition* 24 (2000): 252-258.

Eades, M.R., and M.D. Eades. *Protein Power.* New York: Bantam Books, 1999.

Harper, M.E. "Obesity Research Continues to Spring Leaks." *Clin Invest Med* 20: 239-244.

James, W.P.T., and P. Trayhum. "Thermogenesis and Obesity." *British Medical Bulletin* 37, no. 1 (1981): 43-48.

Juhel, C., M. Armand, Y. Pafumi, et al. "Green Tea Extract (AR25) Inhibits Lipolysis of Triglycerides in Gastric and Duodenal Medium in vitro." *J Nutr Biochem* 11 (2000): 45-51.

Kikutani, T. "Contrary Views on Chinese Herbal Drugs and Side Effects." *International Journal of Oriental Medicine* 15 (1990): 184-188

Kalix, P. "The Pharmacology of Psychotactive Alkaloids from Ephedra and Catha." *J Ethnoparniac* 32, nos. 1-3 (1991): 201-208.

Mills, S.Y., *Essential Book of Herbal Medicine.* London: Penguin, 1991.

Pasquali R., M. Cesari, N. Melchionda, C. Steanini, A. Raitano, and G. Labo. "Does Ephedrine Promote Weight Loss in Low-Energy-Adapted Obese Women?" *International Journal of Obesity* 11 (1987): 163-168.

Pasquali R., M. Cesari, L. Besteghi, N. Melchionda, and V. Balestra. "Thermogenic Agents in the Treatment of Human Obesity: Preliminary Results." *International Journal of Obesity* issue#: 23-26.

Chapter 2:

Atkins, R. Dr. Atkins' New Diet Revolution. New York: M. Evans & Co., 1999.

Borrud, L., C.W. Enns, and S. Mickle. "What We Eat in America: USDA Surveys Food Consumption Changes." *Food Review* 19 (1996): 14-20.

Cassidy, C.M. "Nutrition and Health in Agriculturists and Hunter-Gatherers: A Case Study of Two Prehistoric Populations." *Nutritional Anthropology*, Pleasantville, New York: 117-145.

Calorie Control Council. "Fat Reduction in Foods." *Calorie Control Council Commentary* (1996).

"America: Drowning in Sugar" Experts Call for Food Labels to Disclose Added Sugars. Center For Science in The Public Interest issue date (1999).

Challem, J., et al. *Syndrome X: The Complete Nutritional Program to Prevent and Reverse Insulin Resistance*. New York: John Wiley & Sons, 2001.

Curtis, H. *Biology*. 4th ed. New York: Worth, 1986.

Eades, M.R., and M.D. Eades. *Protein Power*. New York: Bantam, 1999.

Eaton, S.B, et al. "An Evolutionary Perspective Enhances Understanding of Human Nutritional Requirements." *Journal of Nutrition* 126 (1996): 1732-1740.

Eaton, S.B. "Humans, Lipids and Evolution." *Lipids* 27, no. 10 (1992): 814-820.

Galbo, H. "Endocrinology and Metabolism in Exercise." *International Journal of Sports Medicine* 2 (1981): 125.

King, B.J. *Fat Wars: 45 days to Transform Your Body*. Toronto: Macmillan, 2002.

McDowdl, M.A., et al. Energy and Macronutrient Intakes of Persons Ages 2 Months and Over in the United States: Third National Health and Nutrition Examination Survey, Phase 1, 1988-91.

Patterson, C.R. *Essentials of Biochemistry*. London: Pittman, 1983.

Sears, B. *The Anti-Aging Zone*. New York: HarperCollins, 1999.

Scheen, A.J. "From Obesity to Diabetes: Why, When and Who?" *Acta Clin Belg* 55, no. 1 (2000): 9-15.

Taskinen, M.R., and E. Nikkila. "Lipoprotein Lipase of Adipose Tissue and Skeletal Muscle in Human Obesity" *Metabolism* 30 (1981): 810-817.

Yamashita, S., and S. Melmed. "Effects of Insulin on Rat Pituitary Cells: Inhibition of Growth Hormone Secretion and MRNA Levels." *Diabetes* 35 (1986): 440-447.

Yudkin, J. "Evolutionary and Historical Changes in Dietary Carbohydrates." *American Journal of Clinical Nutrition* 20, no. 2 (1967): 108-115.

Chapter 3

Baumel, S. *Serotonin: How to Naturally Harness the Power Behind Prozac and Phen/Fen*. Place: Keats, 1997.

Birdsall, T.C. "Hydroxytryptophan: A Clinically-Effective Serotonin Precursor." *Altern Med Rev.* 3, no. 4 (1998): 271-280.

Bolla, K.I., et al. "Memory Impairment in Abstinent MDMA ("Ecstasy") Users." *Neurology* 51, no. 6 (1998): 1532-1537.

Cummings, D.E., et al. "Plasma Ghrelin Levels after Diet-Induced Weight Loss or Gastric Bypass Surgery." *New England Journal of Medicine* 346 (2002): 1623-1630.

Colgan, M. *Optimum Sports Nutrition*. New York: Advanced Research Press, 1993.

Colgan, M. *The New Nutrition: Medicine for the Millennium*. Apple, 1995.

Colmers, W., et al. "Integration of NPY, AGRP, and Melanocortin Signals in the Hypothalamic Paraventricular Nucleus: Evidence of a Cellular Basis for the Adipostat." *Neuron* 24 (1999): 155-163.

Conley, E. *America Exhausted*. Vitality, 1998.

Dhillo, W.S., and S.R. Bloom. "Hypothalamic Peptides as Drug Targets for Obesity." *Curr Opin Pharmacol.* 1, no. 6 (2001): 651-655.

Germano, C. *Advantra Z: The Natural Way to Lose Weight Safely*. Kensington, 1998.

Groschl, M., et al. "Preanalytical Influences on the Measurement of Ghrelin." *Clin Chem* 48, no. 7 (2002): 1114-1116.

King, B.J., and M.A. Schmidt. *Bio-Age: Ten Steps to A Younger You.* Toronto: Macmillan, 2001.

Klein, S. "The War against Obesity: Attacking a New Front." *American Journal of Clinical Nutrition* 69, no. 6 (1999): 1061-1063.

Leibowitz, S., and T. Kim. "Impact of a Galanin Antagonist on Exogenous Galanin and Natural Patterns of Fat Ingestion." *Brain Research* 599 (1992): 148-152.

Leibowitz, S., et al. "Insulin Plays Role in Controlling Fat Craving." News from The Rockefeller University, New York: 1995.

McGarry, J.D., and D.W. Foster. "Regulation of Hepatic Fatty Acid Production and Ketone Body Production." *Ann Rev Biochem* 49 (1980): 395-420.

Morr, C.V,. and E.Y. Ha. "Whey Protein Concentrates and Isolates: Processing and Functional Properties." *Crit Rev Fod Sci Nutr* 33, no. 6 (1993): 431-476.

Prasad, C. "Food, Mood and Health: A Neurobiologic Outlook." *Braz J Med Biol Res* 31, no. 12 (1998): 1517-1527.

Sapolsky, R. *Why Zebras Don't Get Ulcers.* New York: W.H. Freeman and Company, 1998.

Somer, E., and N.L. Snyderman. *Food and Mood: The Complete Guide to Eating Well and Feeling Your Best.* Owl Books, 1999.

Toornvliet, A.C., et al. "Serotoninergic Drug-Induced Weight Loss in Carbohydrate Craving Obese Patients." *Int J Obes Relat Meb Disord* 20, no. 10 (1996): 917-920.

Wiley, T.S., and B. Formby. *Lights Out: Sleep, Sugar, and Survival.* New York: Simon & Schuster, 2000.

Wurtman, J.J. "Carbohydrate Craving: Relationship Between Carbohydrate Intake and Disorders of Mood." *Drugs* 39, no. 3 (1990): 49-52.

Wurtman, J.J., and S. Suffers. *The Serotonin Solution.* New York: Ballantine, 1997.

Wurtman, R.J., et al. "Brain Serotonin, Carbohydrate-Craving, Obesity and Depression." *Adv Exp Med Biol* 398 (1996): 35-41.

Chapter 4

Crist, D.M., et al. "Body Composition Response to Exogenous GH during Training in Highly Conditioned Adults." *Journal of Applied Physiology* 65, no. 2 (1988): 579-584.

Curtis, H. *Biology*. 4th ed. New York: Worth, 1986.

Dilman, V.M. *The Grand Biological Clock*. Moscow: Mir, 1989.

Jackson F.R., et al. "Oscillating Molecules and Circadian Clock Output Mechanisms." *Molecular Psychiatry* 3, no. 5 (1998): 381-385.

Klatz, R., and C. Kahn. *Grow Young with HGH*. New York: HarperCollins, 1997.

Mass, J.B., M.L. Wherry, et al. *Power Sleep*. New York: Villard Books, 1998.

Rudman, D., et al. "Effects of Human Growth Hormone in Men over 60 Years Old." *New England Journal of Medicine* 323 (1990): 1-6.

Resta O., et al. "Sleep-Related Breathing Disorders, Loud Snoring and Excessive Daytime Sleepiness in Obese Subjects." *International Journal of Obesity* 25, no. 5 (2001): 669-675

Samra, J.S., et al. "Suppression of the Nocturnal Rise in Growth Hormone Reduces Subsequent Lipolysis in Subcutaneous Adipose Tissue." *Eur J Clin Invest* 29, no. 12 (1999): 1045-1052.

Sonntag, W., et al. "Moderate Caloric Restriction Alters the Subcellular Distribution of Somatostatin mRNA and Increases Growth Hormone Pulse Amplitude in Aged Animals." *Neuroendocrinology* 61, no. 5 (1995): 601-608.

Sonntag, W.E., et al. "Pleiotropic Effects of Growth Hormone and Insulin-like Growth Factor (IGF)-1 on Biological Aging: Inferences from Moderate Caloric-restricted Animals." *J Gerontol A Biol Sci Med Sci* 54, no. 12 (1999): B521-538.

Vioque, J., et al. "Time Spent Watching Television, Sleep Duration and Obesity in Adults Living in Valencia, Spain. *International Journal of Obesity* 24, no. 12 (2000): 1683-1688

von Kries, R., et al. "Reduced Risk for Overweight and Obesity in 5- and 6-year-old Children by Duration of Sleep-a Cross-Sectional Study. *International Journal of Obesity* 26, no. 5 (2002): 710-716

Wiley, T.S., and B. Formby. *Lights Out*. New York: Pocket Books, 2000.

Zhang K., et al. "Sleeping Metabolic Rate in Relation to Body Mass Index and Body Composition." *International Journal of Obesity* 26, no. 3 (2002): 376-383

Chapter 5

"Soy May Actually Make Your Thyroid Lazy." *USA Womans World*, 16 March 2001.

Backstrom, T. "Neuroendocrinology of Premenstrual Syndrome." *Clin Obset & Gynecol* 35 (1992): 612.

Barnes, S. "The Chemopreventive Properties of Soy Isoflavonoids in Animal Models of Breast Cancer." *Breast Cancer Res Treat* 46 (1997): 2-3, 169-179.

_____ "Soy Isoflavonoids and Cancer Prevention. Underlying Biochemical and Pharmacological Issues." *Adv Exp Med Biol* 401 (1996): 87-100.

Barnhart, Edward R. *Physicians' Desk Reference*. 45th ed. Oradell, NJ: Medical Economics, 1991.

Baumgartner, R.N., et al. "Associations of Fat and Muscle Masses with Bone Mineral in Elderly Men and Women." *American Journal of Clinical Nutrition* 63. 365.

Bellizi, M.C., and W.H. Dietz. "Workshop on Childhood Obesity: Summary of the Discussion." *American Journal of Clinical Nutrition* 70, supplement (1999): 173S-175S.

Bhasin, S., et al. "The Effects of Supraphysiologic Doses of Testosterone on Muscle Size and Strength in Normal Men." *New England Journal of Medicine* 335, no. 1 (1996): 1-7.

Bouchard, C., et al. "Inheritance of the Amount and Distribution of Human Body Fat." *Int J Obesity* 12 (1998): 205.

Campbell, D.R., and M.S. Kurzer. "Flavonoid Inhibition of Aromatase Enzyme Activity in Human Preadipocytes." *J Steroid Biochem Mol Biol* 46, no. 3 (1993): 381-388.

Caprio, S. et al., "Metabolic Impact of Obesity in Childhood." *Endocrinol Metab Clin North Am* 28, no. 4 (1999): 731-747.

Castleman, M. *The Healing Herbs*. New York: Bantam, 1995.

Cauley, J.A., et al. "The Epidemiology of Serum Sex Hormones in Postmenopausal Women." *Am J Epidem* 129 (1989): 1120.

Cutting, T.M., et al. "Like Mother, Like Daughter: Familial Patterns of Overweight Are Mediated by Mothers' Dietary Disinhibition." *American Journal of Clinical Nutrition* 69, no. 4 (1999): 608-613.

Ferraro, R., et al. "Lower Sedentary Metabolic Rates in Women Compared with Men." *J Clin Invest* 90 (1992): 780.

Fisher, B., et al. "Strength Training Parameters in the Edmonton Police Force Following Supplementation with Elk Velvet Antler (EVA)." (1998).

Futagawa, N.K., et al. "Effect of Age on Body Composition and Resting Metabolic Rate." *Am J Physiol* 259 (1990): E233.

Golan, M.I., et al. "Parents as the Exclusive Agents of Change in the Treatment of Childhood Obesity." *Am J Clin Nutr* 67, no. 6 (1998): 1130-1135.

Hryb, D.J., et al. "The Effect of Extracts of the Roots of the Stinging Nettle (Urtica dioica) on the Interaction of SHBG with Its Receptor on Human Prostatic Membranes" *Planta Med* 61, no. 1 (1995): 31-32.

Hsieh, C., and J. Granstrom. "Staying Young Forever: Putting New Research Findings into Practice." *Life Extension*, December 1999.

Hsieh, C., et al. "Predictors of Sex Hormone Levels Among the Elderly: A Study in Greece." *J of Clin Endocrinology and Metab* 10 (1999): 837-841.

Hsieh, C., and P. Björntorp. "The Interactions between Hypothalamic-Pituitary-Adrenal Axis Activity, Testosterone, Insulin-like Growth Factor I and Abdominal Obesity with Metabolism and Blood Pressure in Men." *Int J Obes Relat Metab Disord* 22, no. 12 (1998): 1184-1196.

Kaym, S., et al. "Associations of Body Mass and Fat Distribution with Sex Hormone Concentrations in Postmenopausal Women." *Int J Epidemiol* (1991): 151.

King, B.J., and M.A. Schmidt. *Bio-Age: Ten Steps to a Younger You*. Toronto: Macmillan, 2001.

Knudsen, C. "Super Soy: Health Benefits of Soy Protein." *Energy Times*, February 1996, p. 12.

Laux, M., and C. Conrad. *Natural Woman, Natural Menopause*. New York: HarperCollins, 1998.

Ley, C.J., et al. "Sex and Menopausal Associated Changes in Body Fat Distribution." *Am J Clin Nutr* 55 (1992): 950.

Mauriège, P,. et al. "Abdominal Fat Cell Lipolysis, Body Fat Distribution, and Metabolic Variables in Premenopausal Women." *J of Clin Endocrinology and Metab* issue, number (1990).

Metzger, B.E., et al. "Amniotic Fluid Insulin Concentration as a Predictor of Obesity" *Arch Dis Child* 65, no. 10 (1990): 1050-1052.

Mindell, E. *Earl Mindell's Soy Miracle*. New York: Simon & Schuster, 1995.

Morgan, P., et al. *The Female Body, An Owner's Manual: A Head to Toe Guide to Good Health and Body Care*. city of publicaton: Rodale Press, 1996.

Pasquali, R., et al. "Body Weight, Fat Distribution and the Menopausal Status in Women." *International Journal of Obesity* 18, no. 9 (1994): 614-621.

Rink, J.D., et al. "Cellular Characterization of Adipose Tissue from Various Body Sites of Women." *J of Clin Endocrinology and Metab* (1996).

Robinson, T.N. "Does Television Cause Childhood Obesity?" *JAMA* 279, no. 12 (1998): 959-960.

Rosenbloom, A.L., et al. "Emerging Epidemic of Type 2 Diabetes in Youth." *Diabetes Care* 22, no. 2 (1999): 345-354.

Rosmond, R., and P. Björntorp. "Endocrine and Metabolic Aberrations in Men with Abdominal Obesity in Relation to Anxio-depressive Infirmity." *Metabolism* 47, no. 10 (1998):1187-1193.

Schöttner, M., et al. "Lignans from the Roots of Urtica dioica and Their Metabolites Bind to Human Sex Hormone Binding Globulin (SHBG)." *Planta Med* 63, no. 6 (1997): 529-532.

Shippen, E., and W. Fryer. *The Testosterone Syndrome: The Critical Factor for Energy, Health and Sexuality*. New York: M. Evans and Company, 1998.

Simpson, E. "Regulation of Estrogen Biosynthesis by Human Adipose Cells." *Endocrin Rev* 10 (1989): 136.

Sothern, M.S., et al. "A Multidisciplinary Approach to the Treatment of Childhood Obesity." *Del Med J* 71, no. 6 (1999): 255-261.

Strauss, R. "Childhood Obesity." *Curr Probl Pediatr* 29, no. 1 (1999): 1-29.

Swartz, C. "Low Serum Testosterone: A Cardiovascular Risk in Elderly Men." *Geriatric Med Today* 7, no. 12 (1998).

Tchernof, A., et al. "Relationships between Endogenous Steroid Hormone, Sex Hormone-Binding Globulin and Lipoprotein Levels in Men: Contribution of Visceral Obesity, Insulin Levels and Other Metabolic Variables." *Atherosclerosis* 133, no. 2 (year): 235-244.

Vermeulen, A., et al. "Testosterone, Body Composition and Aging." *J Endocrinol Invest* 22, no. 5 (1999): 110-116.

Volek, J.S., et al. "Testoserone and Cortisol in Relationship to Dietary Nutrients and Resistance Exercise." *Journal of Applied Physiology* 82, no. 1 (1997): 49-54.

Walker, M. "Concentrated Soybean Phytochemicals." *Healthy & Natural Journal* 2, no. 2 (1994): page refs.

"Phytochemicals in Soybeans." *Health Foods Business*, March 1995, p. 36.

Waterhouse, D. *Outsmarting the Midlife Fat Cell*. New York: Hyperion, 1998.

Wright, J., and L. Lenard. *Maximize Your Vitality and Potency: For Men over 40.* Petaluma: Smart Publications, 1999.

Zamboni, M., et al. "Body Fat Distribution in Pre and Post-menopausal Women: Metabolic and Antropometric Variables in the Interrelationships." *Int J Obesity* 16 (1992): 495.

Zeligs, M.A. "Plant-Powered Weight Loss: Phytonutrition for a Fat-Burning Metabolism." (2001).

Chapter 6

American Heart Association http://www.americanheart.org

Baba, N.H., et al. "High Protein vs. High Carbohydrate Hypoenergetic Diet for the Treatment of Obese Hyperinsulinemic Subjects." *Int J Obes Relat Metab Disord* 23, no. 11 (1999): 1202-1206.

Ballerini, R. "Double-Blind, Placebo-Controlled Study of 60 Human Subjects." Milano, Italy, Sept. 7, 2001.

Barenys, M., et al. "Effect of Exercise and Protein Intake on Energy Expenditure in Adolescents." *Rev Esp Fisiol* 49, no. 4 (1993): 209-217.

Batmanghelidj, F. *Your Body's Many Cries for Water.* 2nd ed.: Global Health Solutions, 1997.

Behall, K.M., D.J. Scholfield, and J. Hallfrisch. "Effect of Beta-glucan Level in Oat Fiber Extracts on Blood Lipids in Men and Women." *J. Am. Coll.* Nutr 16 (1997): 46-51.

Berry, E.M. "Dietary Fatty Acids in the Management of Diabetes Mellitus." *Am J Clin Nutr* 66 (1997): 991S-997S.

Biolo, G., et al. "An Abundant Supply of Amino-Acids Enhances the Metabolic Effect of Exercise on Muscle Protein." *Amer J Phys* 273 (1997): E122-E129.

Blankson, H., et al. "Conjugated Linoleic Acid Reduces Body Fat Mass in Overweight and Obese Humans." *J Nutr* 130, no. 12 (2000): 2943-2948.

Bonora, E., et al. "Impaired Glucose Tolerance, Type II Diabetes Mellitus and Carotid Atherosclerosis: Prospective Results from the Bruneck Study." *Diabetologia* 43, no. 2 (2000): 156-164.

Borkman, M., et al. "The Relationship Between Insulin Sensitivity and the Fatty-Acid Composition of Skeletal-Muscle Phospholipids." *New England Journal of Medicine* 328, no. 4 (1993): 238-244.

Bounous, G. and P. Gold. "The Biological Activity of Undenatured Dietary Whey Proteins: Role of Glutathione." *Clin Invest Med* 14, no. 4 (1991): 296-309.

Bounous, G., et al. "Evolutionary Traits in Human Milk Proteins." *Med Hypotheses* 27, no. 2 (1998): 133-140.

Bourden, I., W. Yokoyama, P. Davis, C. Hudson, R. Backus, D. Richter, B. Knuckles, and B. Schneeman. "Postprandial Lipid, Glucose, Insulin and Cholecystokinin Responses in Men Fed Barley Pasta Enriched with Beta-glucan." *Am. J. Clin. Nutr* 69 (1999): 55-63.

Brand, J.C., S. Colagiuri, S. Corssman, A. Allen, D.C.K. Roberts, and A.S. Truswell. "Low-Glycemic Index Foods Improve Longterm Glycemic Control in NIDDM." *Diabetes Care* 14 (1991): 95-101.

Broadhurst, C.L. "Balanced Intakes of Natural Triglycerides for Optimum Nutrition: An Evolutionary and Phytochemical Perspective." *Med Hypotheses* 49, no. 3 (1997): 247-261.

Campbell, W.W., et al. "Effects of an Omnivorous Diet Compared with a Lactoovovegetarian Diet on Resistance-Training-Induced Changes in Body Composition and Skeletal Muscle in Older Men." *Am J Clin Nutr* 70 (1999): 1032-1039.

Cassidy, C.M. "Nutrition and Health in Agriculturalists and Hunter-Gatherers: A Case Study of Two Prehistoric Populations." Nutr Anth: Pleasantville, New York: Pedgrave: 117-145.

Conley, E. *America Exhausted*. Flint: Vitality Press, 1998.

Coyne, L.L. *Fat Won't Make You Fat*. Fish Creek Publishing, 1998.

Crayhon, R. "The Paleolithic Diet and Its Modern Implications An Interview with Loren Cordain, PhD." *Life Service Supplement News*, 26 July, 1999.

Demmelmair, H., et al. "Trans Fatty Acid Contents in Spreads and Cold Cuts Usually Consumed by Children." *Z Ernahrungswiss* 35, no. 3 (1996): 235-240.

Dreon, D.M., et al. "A Very Low-Fat Diet Is Not Associated with Improved Lipoprotein Profiles in Men with a Predominance of Large, Low-density Lipoproteins." *Am J Clin Nutr* 69, no. 3 (1999): 411-418.

Froyland, L., et al. "Mitochondrion Is the Principal Target for Nutritional and Pharmacological Control of Triglyceride Metabolism." *J Lipid Res* 38, no. 9 (1997): 1851-1858.

Garg, A. "High-Monounsaturated-Fat Diets for Patients with Diabetes Mellitus: A Meta-analysis." *Am J Clin Nutr* 67, no. 3 (1998): 577S-582S.

Garg, A., et al. "Effects of Varying Carbohydrate Content of Diet in Patients with Non-insulin-dependent Diabetes Mellitus." *JAMA* 271, no. 18 (1994): 1421-1428.

Gimeno, E., et al. "Effect of Ingestion of Virgin Olive Oil on Human Low-density Lipoprotein Composition." *Eur J Clin Nutr* 56, no. 2 (2002): 114-120

Gittleman, A.L. *The 40-30-30 Phenomenon*. Keats Publishing, 1997.

Glore, S.R., D. Van Treeck, A.W. Knehans, and M. Guild. "Soluble Fiber and Serum Lipids: a Literature Review." *J. Am. Diet*. Assoc 94 (1994): 425-436.

Golay, A., et al. "Weight-loss with Low or High Carbohydrate Diet?" *Int J Obes Relat Metab Disord* 20, no. 12 (1996): 1067-1072.

Grant, W.B. "Low-fat, High-sugar Diet and Lipoprotein Profiles." *Am J Clin Nutr* 70, no. 6 (1999): 1111-1112.

Harnack, L., et al. "Soft Drink Consumption Among U.S. Children and Adolescents: Nutritional Consequences." *J Am Diet Assoc* 4 (1999): 436-441.

Harris, W.S., et al. "Influence of n-3 Fatty Acid Supplementation on the Endogenous Activities of Plasma Lipase." *Am J Clin Nutr* 66, no. 2 (1997): 254-260.

Heleniak, E., and B. Aston. "Prostaglandins, Brown Fat and Weight Loss." *Med Hypoth* 28 (1989): 13-33.

Ink, S., and R. Matthews. "Oatmeal and Oat-bran: Heart Healthy Benefits and More," *New Technologies for Healthy Foods and Nutraceuticals*, ed. M. Yalpani. Shrewsbury: ATL Press, 1997.

Jenkins, D.J.A., T.M.S. Wolever, A.R. Leeds, M.A. Gassull, P. Haisman, J. Dilawari, D.V. Goff, G.L. Metz, and K.G.M.M. Alberti. "Dietary Fibres, Fiber Analogues, and Glucose Tolerance: Importance of Viscosity." *Br. Med. J* 1 (1978): 1392-1394.

Judd, P.A., and A.S. Trusswell. "The Effect of Rolled Oats on Blood Lipids and Fecal Steroid Excretion in Man." *Am. J. Clin. Nutr* 34 (1981): 2061-2067.

King, B.J., and M.A. Schmidt. *Bio-Age: Ten Steps to a Younger You*. Toronto: Macmillan, 2001.

Kinosian, B.P., and Eisenberg, J.M. "Cutting into Cholesterol. Cost-Effective Alternatives for Treating Hypercholetserolemia." *JAMA* 259 (1988): 2249-2254.

Knudsen, C. "Super Soy: Health Benefits of Soy Protein." *Energy Times*, February 1996, p. 12.

Kwiterovich, P.O., Jr. "The Effect of Dietary Fat, Antioxidants, and Pro-Oxidants on Blood Lipids, Lipoproteins, and Atherosclerosis." *J Am Diet Assoc* 7 (1997): S31-S41.

Lardinois, C.K. "The Role of Omega-3 Fatty Acids on Insulin Secretion and Insulin Sensitivity." *Med Hypotheses* 24, no. 3 (1987): 243-248.

Lavin, J.H., et al. "The Effect of Sucrose and Aspartame Sweetened Drinks on Energy Intake, Hunger, and Food Choice of Female, Moderately Restrained Eaters." *Int J Obes Relat Metab Disord* 21, no. 1 (1997): 37-42.

Lemon, P.W., et al. "Moderate Physical Activity Can Increase Dietary Protein Needs." *Can J Appl Physiol* 22, no. 5 (1997): 494-503.

Louheranta, A.M., et al. "A High-Trans Fatty Acid Diet and Insulin Sensitivity in Young Healthy Women." *Metabolism*, 48, no. 7 (1999): 870-875.

Marlett, J.A., K.B. Josig, N.W. Vollendorf, F.L. Shinnick, V.S. Haack, and J.A. Story. "Mechanism of Serum Cholesterol Reduction by Oat Bran." *Hepatology* 20 (1994): 1450-1457.

McCrory, M.A., et al. "Overeating in America: Association Between Restaurant Food Consumption and Body Fatness in Healthy Adult Men and Women Ages 19 to 80." *Obes Res* 7, no. 6 (1999): 564-571.

Miller, J.C. "Importance of Glycemic Index in Diabetes." *Am J Clin Nutr* 59 (1994): 747S-752S.

Mindell, E. *Earl Mindell's Soy Miracle*. Simon & Schuster, 1995.

Mock, D.M. "Marginal Biotin Deficiency During Normal Pregnancy." *Am J Clin Nutr* 75, no. 2 (2002): 295-299

Morr, C.V., and E.Y. Ha. "Whey Protein Concentrates and Isolates: Processing and Functional Properties." *Crit Rev Food Sci Nutr* 33, no. 6 (1993): 431-476.

Nelson, G.J., P.C. Schmidt, and D.S. Kelly. "Low-fat Diets Do Not Lower Plasma Cholesterol Levels in Healthy Men Compared to High-fat Diets with Similar Fatty Acid Composition at Constant Calorie Intake." *Lipids* 30, no. 11 (1995): 969-976.

Pick, M.E., Z.J. Hawrysh, M.I. Gee, E. Toth, M.L. Garg, and R.T. Hardin. "Oat Bran Concentrate Bread Products Improve Longterm Control of Diabetes: a Pilot Study." *J. Am. Diet.* Assoc 96 (1996): 1254-1261.

Ramadasan, K., and R.C. Srimal. "LD 50 Acute Toxicity Study." Amala Cancer Research Center, Trichur, India, April 29, 2002.

Reaven, G.M. "Do High Carbohydrate Diets Prevent the Development or Attenuate the Manifestations (Or Both) of Syndrome X? A Viewpoint Strongly Against." *Curr Opin Lipidol* 8, no.1 (1997): 23-27.

Reaven, G.M., and C. Hollenbeck. "Variation of Insulin Stimulated Glucose Uptake in Healthy Individuals with Normal Glucose Tolerance." *J Clin Endocrinol Metab* 64 (1987): 1169-1173.

Riserus, U., et al. "Conjugated Linoleic Acid (CLA) Reduced Abdominal Adipose Tissue in Obese Middle-aged Men with Signs of the Metabolic Syndrome: A Randomized Controlled Trial." *Int J Obes Relat Metab Disord* 25, no. 8 (2001): 1129-1135.

Robinson, S.M., et al. "Protein Turnover and Thermogenesis in Response to High-Protein and High-Carbohydrate Feeding in Men." *Am J Clin Nutr* 52, no. 1 (1990): 72-80.

Rossner, S. "Dietary Fiber in the Prevention and Treatment of Obesity," *Dietary Fibre, A Component of Food: Nutritional Function in Health and Disease*, ed. T.F. Schweizer and C.A. Edwards. New York: Springer-Verlag, 1992.

Rustan, A.C., et al. "Omega-3 and Omega-6 Fatty Acids in the Insulin Resistance Syndrome." *Ann NY Acad Sci* 20, no. 827 (1997): 310-326.

Satterlee, L.D., et al. "In Vitro Assay for Predicting Protein Efficiency Ratio as Measured by Rat Bioassay: Collaborative Study." *J Assoc Off Anal Chem* Jul 65, no. 4 (1982): 798-809.

Schmidt, M.A. *Smart Fats*. Berkeley: North Atlantic Books, 1997.

Sears, B. *The Anti-Aging Zone*. New York: HarperCollins, 1999.

Sidossis, L.S., et al. "Glucose Plus Insulin Regulates Fat Oxidation by Controlling the Rate of Fatty Acid Entry into the Mitochondria." *J Clin Invest* 98, no. 10 (1996): 2244-2250.

Simoneau, J.A., et al. "Markers of Capacity to Utilize Fatty Acids in Human Skeletal Muscle: Relation to Insulin Resistance and Obesity and Effects of Weight Loss." *FASEB J* 13, no. 14(1999): 2051-2060.

Simopoulos, A.P. "Is Insulin Resistance Influenced by Dietary Linoleic Acid and Trans Fatty Acids?" *Free Radic Biol Med* 17, no. 4 (1994): 367-372.

Simopoulos, A.P. "Evolutionary Aspects of Nutrition and Health: Diet, Exercise, Genetics and Chronic Disease." *World Review of Nutrition and Dietetics*, vol. 84. S. Karger, 1999.

Soucy, J., and J. Leblanc. "Protein Meals and Postprandial Thermogenesis." *Physiol Behav* 65 (1999): 4-5.

Vandewater, K. and Z. Vickers. "Higher-Protein Foods Produce Greater Sensory-Specific Satiety." *Physiol Behav* 59, no. 3 (1996): 579-583.

Vinson, J.A. and D.M. Shuta. "Double Blind, Placebo-Controlled, Cross-Over Pilot Study of 11 Adult Human Subjects Which Showed 66% Less Starch Absorption in the Group Taking Phase 2." Department of Chemistry, University of Scranton, April 24, 2002.

Whitehead, J.M., et al. "The Effect of Protein Intake on 24-Hour Energy Expenditure During Energy Restriction." *Int J Obes Relat Metab Disord* 20, no. 8 (1996): 727-732.

Willett, W.C., et al. "Is Dietary Fat a Major Determinant of Body Fat?" *Am J Clin Nutr* 67 (1998): 556S-562S.

Wursch, P., and F.X. Pi-Sunyer. "The Role of Viscous Soluble Fiber in the Metabolic Control of Diabetes. *Diabetes Care* 20 (1997): 1774-1780.

Wolfe, B.M., and L.A. Piche. "Replacement of Carbohydrate by Protein in a Conventional-fat Diet Reduces Cholesterol and Triglyceride Concentrations in Healthy Normo-lipidemic Subjects." *Clin Invest Med* 22, no. 4 (1999): 140-148.

Zed, C., and W.P. James. "Dietary Thermogenesis in Obesity. Response to Carbohydrate and Protein Meals: The Effect of Beta-Adrenergic Blockage and Semi-Starvation." *Int J Obes* 10, no. 5 (1986): 391-405.

"Battling Body Fat With CLA"
Boxed Text References, Chapter 6, page 70

Benito, P., Nelson, G.J., Kelley, D.S., Bartolini, G., Schmidt, P.C., Simon, V. "The Effect of Conjugated Linoleic Acid on Plasma Lipoproteins and Tissue Fatty Acid Composition in Humans." *Lipids*. 36:229-236 (2001).

Clouet, P., Demizieux, L., Gresti, J., Degrace, P. "Mitochondrial Respiration on Rumenic and Linoleic Acids." *Biochem. Soc. Trans.* 29(Part 2):320-325 (2001).

Devery, R., Miller, A., Stanton, C. "Conjugated Linoleic Acid and Oxidative Behaviour in Cancer Cells." *Biochem. Soc. Trans.* 29(Part 2):341-344 (2001).

Kritchevsky, D., Czarnecki S.K. "Conjugated Linoleic Acid (CLA) in Health and Disease." *Chim. Oggi* (Chemistry Today) 19(6):26-28 (2001).

Lawson, R.E., Moss. A.R., Givens, D.I. "The Role of Dairy Products in Supplying Conjugated Linoleic Acid to Man's Diet: A Review." *Nutr. Res. Rev.* 14:153-172 (2001).

Rahman, S.M., Wang, Y.M., Han, S.Y., Cha, J.Y., Fukuda, N., Yotsumoto, H., Yanagita, T. "Effects of Short-Term Administration of Conjugated Linoleic Acid on Lipid Metabolism in White and Brown Adipose Tissues of Starved/Refed Otsuka Long-Evans Tokushima Fatty Rats." *Food Res. Int.* 34:515-520 (2001).

Roche, H.M., Noone, E., Nugent, A., Gibney, M.J. "Conjugated Linoleic Acid: A Novel Therapeutic Nutrient." *Nutr. Res. Rev.* 14:173-187 (2001).

Suzuki, R., Noguchi, R., Ota, T., Abe, M., Miyashita, K., Kawada, T. "Cytotoxic Effect of Conjugated Trienoic Fatty Acids on Mouse Tumor and Human Monocytic Leukemia Cells." *Lipids.* 36:477-482 (2001).

INDEX

A

abdominal crunches on ball, 214
abdominal exercises, 213–215
abst+, 219
addiction to food, 34
adenosine triphosphate (ATP),
    14, 77
adrenaline, 30
Adrogel, 51
AdvantraZ™, 16
aerobic activity, 49, 176, 177
    see also Biocize
aging, 77
alpha amylase, 74–75
alpha-linolenic acid (ALA). *See*
    omega-3 fatty acids
*American Journal of Clinical
    Nutrition*, 16, 33
amino acids, 45, 62
anabolism, 61
ancestors, 17–18, 70
Androderm, 51
androgens, 48
anti-craving formulas, 220–221
apple fiber, 123
arm exercises, 215–216
aromatase, 50
arugula, 122

asparagus omelette with bagel,
    133
ATP (adenosine triphosphate), 14
avidin, 64

B

back exercises, 210–212
ball squat on wall, 208
banana chocolate shake, 132
banana peach shake, 133
barbell bench press, 203
Batmanghelidj, F., 77
beans, 59
bee pollen, 122
beef. *See* meats
beginners, 109–110
bent over row, 210
berries, 121, 122
berry cottage cheese, 148
berry orange, 156
berry shake, 131
beta-3 receptors, 15
beta-endorphins, 31, 100–101
beta-glucan, 82–83
beverages and shakes
    banana chocolate shake, 132
    banana peach shake, 133
    berry orange, 156

berry shake, 131
blueberry shake-it, 142
carrot top shake, 139
chocolate dreams, 157
colada, frozen, 145
cran-apple fun, 162
frozen blue, 159
green beret, 160
holiday shake, 137
kiwi-banana rama, 152
orchard blend, 144
phytonutrient delight, 151
protein boost, 135
protein dream, 154
protein punch, 146
protein rush, 140
strawberry/rhubarb shake, 150
sweet and sour shake, 141
Tahiti treat, 165
veggie protein surprise, 163
yogurt delight, 147
biceps curls, 215
bioavailable growth factors, 45
Biocize
    see also exercise
    advanced exercisers, 192
    anabolism, 176–178
    beginners, 191–192

best time for, 182
drop sets, 192–193
duration of exercise, 179
eating after, 183
eating before, 182–183
equipment, 175–176
gasping, 178–179
goal of, 174
introduction, 173–175
optimum duration of cardio,
    179–180
optimum duration of resist-
    ance exercise, 180
phase I program, 194–196
phase II program, 196–198
phase III program, 199–202
resistance, 191
resting phase, 193
rules, 184
sets and repetitions, 187–189,
    190–191
tempo, 189–191
timing of cardio, 180
and travel, 185–186
Biocize exercises
    abdominal section, 213–215
    arm section, 215–216
    back section, 210–212
    chest section, 203–204
    leg section, 207–209
    shoulder section, 205–207
biological ancestry, 17–18, 70
biological clocks, 40
Bisphenol A (BPA), 5
blueberry shake-it, 142
body fat
    aromatase, 50
    Body Mass Index (BMI), 8–9
    fat cells. See fat cells
    general body fat percentage
        categories, 8
    men's, 48–51
    methods of measurement, 8–9
    vs. muscle, 7
    stored, 12
    and thermogenesis, 15

waist circumference, 9
    vs. weight, 6–7
    women's, 51–57
Body Mass Index (BMI), 8–9
borage oil, 123–124
bovine colostrum, 45
Bowman Gray School of Medi-
    cine, 45
breads, 124–125
British Journal of Public Health, 2
broccoli, 122
broccoli soup, 147
broccoli sprouts, 122
Brookhaven National
    Laboratory, 34
brown rice, 123
burrito, 142
butter, vs. margarine, 128–129

C
cabbage, 122
caffeine, 75–76, 78
Cajun cod, 166
calcium, 126–127
calories, 60
carbohydrates
    beta-endorphons, 31
    break-down of, 72
    eating principles, 115
    glycemic index, 73–74
    high-carbohydrate diets,
        36–37
    high-glycemic, 72
    and insulin, 20
    low-glycemic, 33, 72
    necessary daily amounts,
        21–22
    vs. protein, 62
    and serotonin, 31–32
cardiovascular disease, 3
carrot top shake, 139
catabolism, 61
catechins, 16
cauliflower, 122
cheese whiz, 149
chest exercises, 203–204

chicken sandwich, 147
chicken soup, 152
chicken wrap, 162
childhood obesity
    prevalence, 57
    sleep, effect of, 39
    Type II diabetes, 57
chili, 135
chocolate dreams, 157
cholecystokinin (CCK), 35, 96
chrysin, 50
chrysin with piperine extract, 223
Citrus aurantium, 15
citrus fruits, 121
cod, Cajun, 166
colada, frozen, 145
cold-water fish and fish oils,
    123–124
Colorado State University, 73
colostrum, 221–222
conjugated linoleic acid (CLA),
    68–70, 225–226
container choices, 5
cooked oats, organic, 130
Cordain, Loren, 73
Cornell University, 39
cortisol, 30, 90–91
cran-apple fun, 162
cravings, 30–32, 33–34

D
daily caloric needs, 109
Daily Total Fat Wars Recom-
    mended Macronutrient Break-
    down Chart, 113–114
dead lift, 211
diabetes
    Type I, 22
    Type II. See Type II diabetes
Diabetes Care, 83
dietary fats
    bad fats, 66–67
    conjugated linoleic acid
        (CLA), 68–70
    eating principles, 116
    essential fatty acids, 67–68

good fats, 65–66
monounsaturated fats (MUFA), 66
necessity of, 64–65
polyunsaturated fats, 66
saturated fats, 66–67
trans fats, 67
unsaturated fats, 65
diets
common variations, 36–37
and cravings, 30–32
high-carbohydrate, 36–37
high-protein, 37
low-calorie, 36
muscle, enemy of, 29
and nutrient deprivation, 33
unsuccessful, 27–28
dihydrotestosterone (DHT), 49
diindolylmethane (DIM), 56
dopamine, 34, 40, 98–99
dressings. See salads and dressings
drop sets, 192–193
dumbbell bench press, 204
dumbbell lunge, 209

E
Eades, Dan, 12
Eades, Mary, 12
eating out, 167–171
eating principles, 115–116
Eaton, Boyd, 17, 18
eggs
asparagus omelette with bagel, 133
benefits of, 125
burrito, 142
egg breakfast, 143–144
egg salad sandwich, 157
free-range, 71
grass-fed, 71
open-faced egg muffin, 138
organic, 126
poached eggs 'n' cheese, 156
raw, 64
spinach and feta eggs, 153
elk velvet antler (EVA), 49

endocrine hormones, 24–25
energy
and ATP (adenosine triphosphate), 14
basic sources of, 43–44
ephedra, 15
essential fatty acids, 67–68, 128, 226–227
estrogen
decline of, 52
diet and exercise, 53
good vs. bad, 56
and men, 50
production of, 52
and soy, 54–55
summary of, 93–94
vs. testosterone, 52
and vegetables, 56
estrogen-replacement therapy (ERT), 54
exercise
see also Biocize; Biocize exercises
aerobic activity, 49, 176, 177
calories burned during activity charge, 181
daily activity, 186
resistance training, 49, 175, 176, 177

F
fat cells
and galanin, 32
how they work, 11–12
number of, 11
and stress, 30
women vs. men, 51
fats. See body fat; dietary fats
fermented soy products, 55
fiber
beta-glucan, 82–83
classes of, 78
insoluble, 79
and insulin, 79–80
role of, 78
soluble, 79

sources of, 80–82
filtered water, 120
fish and seafood
Cajun cod, 166
salmon and stuffed pepper, 158
salmon delight, 138
scallop jambalaya, 152–153
shrimp and miso, 164–165
shrimp salad, 160
shrimp stir-fry, 143
sole, baked, with coleslaw, 132
tuna sandwich, 149
tuna with Greek salad, 148
Fitzpatrick, Michael, 55
flaxseed and flaxseed oil, 122, 123–124, 127
Formby, Bent, 42
Frankenstein fat, 67
free-range meat and eggs, 71, 123, 127
front squat, 207
frozen blue, 159
fruit salad with cottage cheese, 137
fruits
benefits, 123
berry cottage cheese, 148
consumption of variety, 121
recommended list of, 121–124

G
galanin, 32, 101
game meats, 123, 127
garlic, 122
Genetic Nutritioneering (Bland), 6
genetically modified foods, 56
ghrelin, 34
glucagon, 19, 23–24, 87
glycemic index, 73–74, 116–120
glycogen, 21–22
glycomacropeptides (GMPs), 35
granola with strawberries, 141
grapefruit, 155
grapes, 121, 122
grass-fed meat and eggs, 71, 123,

127, 228–229
Greek salad, with tuna, 148
green beret, 160
green-food concentrates, 122
green tea, 16, 122
growth hormone stimulators, 45

H
hamstring curl with ball, 209
hanging row, 210
Hawaiian pineapple delight, 136
hemp oil, 123–124
HGH segretagogues, 222
high alphalactabumin whey iso-
    lates. *See*
    whey-protein isolates
high-carbohydrate diets, 36–37
high-glycemic carbohydrates, 72,
    119–120
high-protein diets, 37
holiday shake, 137
honey miso dressing, 134
hormone metabolism, 56
hormone-sensitive lipase (HSL),
    23–24
hormones
    adrenaline, 30
    androgens, 48
    beta-endorphins, 31, 100–101
    cholecystokinin (CCK), 35, 96
    cortisol, 30, 90–91
    dopamine, 98–99
    endocrine, 24–25
    estrogen. *See* estrogen
    galanin, 32, 101
    ghrelin, 34
    glucagon, 23–24, 87
    human growth hormones
    (HGH), 42–45, 87–88
    importance of, 19
    insulin. *See* insulin
    leptin, 96–97
    melatonin, 41–42, 89
    neuropeptide NPY, 102
    noradrenaline, 99–100

norepinephrine, 99–100
progesterone, 94–95
prolactin, 89–90
serotonin, 31–32, 33, 97–98
sex, 40–41
stress, 40–41
testosterone. *See* testosterone
human growth hormones
    (HGH), 42–45, 87–88, 174
hunter-gatherers, 17–18, 72–73
hypoglycmic episodes, 32
hypothyroidism, 24–25

I
incline dumbbell bench press,
    204
indole-3-carbinol (I3C), 56
insatiable cravings, 30–32
insoluble fiber, 79
insomnia, 42
insulin
    and fiber, 79–80
    process described, 19, 20–21,
    32
    resistance, 23
    summary of, 86
insulin-like growth factors (IGF),
    43, 44
International Journal of Obesity,
    39, 40, 68

J
*Journal of Clinical Endocrinology
    and Metabolism*, 49
Journal of Lipid Research, 5
Journal of Nutrition, 68
junk food, 5

K
kale, 122
kidney beans, 74–75
kiwi-banana rama, 152

L
lamb with wild rice, 150–151

The Lancet, 34
last meal of day, 110
lateral raises, 207
Lauda, Carmen M., 74
lean+, 218–219
lean body mass, 114
leg exercises, 207–209
legumes, 60, 123
leptin, 96–97
lettuce, 122
Lights Out (Wiley and Formby),
    42
linoleic acid (LA). *See* omega-6
    fatty acids
liquid candy, 75–76
low-calorie diets, 36
    see also diets
low-glycemic carbohydrates, 33,
    72, 116–117
lower abdominal leg raises, 215

M
Ma huang, 15
macronutrient breakdown chart,
    113–114
macronutrients, 59
mandarin/chicken salad, 140
margarine, vs. butter, 128–129
Marshall, J. John, 74
Mass, James, 42
meal timing, 110
meats
    chicken sandwich, 147
    chicken soup, 152
    chicken wrap, 162
    game, 123, 127
    grass-fed (free-range), 71, 123,
    127, 228–229
    lamb with wild rice, 150–151
    mandarin/chicken salad, 140
    Mexican marvel, 144–145
    roast beef sandwich, 139
    roasted turkey sandwich, 131
    steak, 60
    steak and yams, 161

steak dinner, 145
steak kabob, 155
melatonin, 41–42, 89
men
  estrogen levels, rise in, 50
  stress and, 50
  testosterone. *see* testosterone
menus
  day 1, 130–132
  day 2, 133–135
  day 3, 136–138
  day 4, 138–140
  day 5, 141–143
  day 6, 143–145
  day 7, 146–148
  day 8, 148–151
  day 9, 151–153
  day 10, 153–155
  day 11, 156–158
  day 12, 159–161
  day 13, 161–163
  day 14, 164–166
  vegetarian food swaps,
    166–167
metabolism, 13–14
Mexican marvel, 144–145
micronutrients, 59
milk and milk products
  see also beverages and shakes
  benefits of, 126
  berry cottage cheese, 146
  cheese whiz, 149
  fruit salad with cottage cheese,
    137
  organic yogurt, 123
  pizza, 154
  poached eggs 'n' cheese, 156
  yogurt delight, 147
  yogurt fruit salad, 161
miso, 122
moderate glycemic foods,
  118–119
modified pull-up, 211
monounsaturated fats (MUFA),
  66

movies, 172
muesli, organic, 136
muesli delight, 148
muscle, 28–29
the muse, 164

N
napping, 42
National Institutes of Health, 39
National Soft Drink Association,
  75
neuropeptide NPY, 102
New England Journal of Medicine,
  34, 43
night shift workers, 110
noradrenaline, 99–100
norepinephrine, 99–100
nutrient deprivation, 33
nuts, 59, 123, 127

O
oat beta-glucans, 228
oat bran, 123
oatmeal, 123
obesity
  biological mechanisms under-
    lying, 5
  complications pf, 2–4
  epidemic, 2
  prevalence, 2
  and testosterone, 48
obstructive sleep apnea (OSA), 44
Ohio State University, 62
omega-3 fatty acids, 66–67, 70,
  127
omega-6 fatty acids, 66–67, 70,
  127
one armed row, 212
onions, 122
open-faced egg muffin, 138
orchard blend, 144
organic foods
  cooked oats, 130
  milk products, 123
  muesli, 136

recommended, 229–230
whole foods, 120–121
yogurt, 123
overhead triceps extension, 216

P
Paleolithic nutrition, 73
peanut butter and banana sandwich, 151
peppers, 122
perimenopause, 52
Pharmachem Laboratories,
  74–75
Phaseolamin 2250, 227–228
phytoestrogens, 54–55
phytonutrient delight, 151
pineapple delight, 136
pizza, 154
poached eggs 'n' cheese, 156
polyphenols, 16
polyunsaturated fats, 66
portions and sizes, 110–111
poultry. *See* meats
prehuman hunter-gatherers,
  17–18, 72–73
progesterone, 94–95
prolactin, 89–90
prolactin production, 41–42
protein
  and beans, 59
  best sources, 63–64
  vs. carbohydrates, 62
  eating principles, 115–116
  and muscle development, 63
  necessity of, 61–63
  and nuts, 59
  and steak, 60
  synthesis, 62
  and testosterone levels, 49
  and thermic value, 15
protein boost, 135
protein dream, 154
Protein Power (Eades and Eades),
  12
protein punch, 146

protein rush, 140
psychological problems, and obesity, 4

R
RAND Institute, 2
raw eggs, 64
red wine, 121
refined foods, 5
repetitions and sets, 187–189, 190–191
resistance, 191
resistance training, 49, 175, 176, 177
    see also Biocize
restaurant eating, 167–171
resting metabolic rate (RMR), 40
roast beef sandwich, 139
roasted turkey sandwich, 131
roll-out, 213
Romanian dead lift, 212
rotator cuff external rotation, 206
rotator cuff internal rotation, 205
Rudman, Daniel, 43

S
salads and dressings
    fruit salad with cottage cheese, 137
    Greek salad, with tuna, 148
    honey miso dressing, 134
    spinach salad, 134
    yogurt fruit salad, 161
salmon and stuffed pepper, 158
salmon delight, 138
salmonella, 126
Sansum Medical Research Institute, 39, 42
saturated fats, 66–67
scallop jambalaya, 152–153
seafood. *See* fish and seafood
secretagogues, 45
seeds, 60, 123, 127
self-evaluation, 106–108

serotonin, 31–32, 33, 97–98
sets and repetitions, 187–189, 190–191
7-grain hot cereal, 159
sex-hormone-binding globulin (SHBG), 48, 49
sex hormones, 40–41
shakes. *See* beverages and shakes
shallots, 122
shoulder exercises, 205–207
shoulder press, 205
shrimp and miso, 164–165
shrimp salad, 160
shrimp stir-fry, 143
side raise to 45 degrees, 206
sleep
    and cravings, reducing, 33
    full sleep cycle, 42
    hormonal schedule, 40–42
    human growth hormones (HGH), 42–45
    melatonin, 41–42
    napping, 42
    necessity of, 39
sleeping metabolic rate (SMR), 40
soft drinks, 75–76
sole, baked, with coleslaw, 132
soluble fiber, 79
somatomedins, 43
somatotrophes, 45
Sonntag, William, 45
soy
    fermented soy products, 55
    genetically modified, 56
    soy sprouts, 122
    soybeans, 122
    and thyroid gland, 55
    and women, 54–55
soy-based protein shakes, 55–56
soy protein isolates, 122, 224
spinach, 122
spinach and feta eggs, 153
spinach salad, 134

sprouts, 122
Stanford University School of Medicine, 3
starch blocker, 227
starch digestion, controlled reduction of, 74–75
steak, 60
steak and yams, 161
steak dinner, 145
steak kabob, 155
stinging nettle root, 50, 222–223
strategy, 111–113
strawberry/rhubarb shake, 150
stress
    and fat, 29–30
    hormones, 40–41
    and serotonin, 33
    and testosterone levels, 50
sumo squat, 208
superman, 214
sweet and sour shake, 141
sweet potatoes, 122
Syndrome X, 22–23

T
Tahiti treat, 165
tea, 16
teen obesity
    prevalence, 57
    Type II diabetes, 57
tempeh, 122
tempo, 189–191
Testoderm, 51
testosterone
    declining levels, 48
    vs. estrogen, 52
    importance of, 48, 174
    and muscle development, 52
    obesity, direct inverse relationship with, 48
    replacement, 51
    restoration of, 48–49
    and stress, 50
    summary of, 91–92